Defeat
Chronic Fatigue Syndrome:

You Don't Have to Live With It

Defeat

··

Chronic Fatigue Syndrome:

You Don't Have to Live With It

AN EIGHT STEP PROTOCOL

Martha E. Kilcoyne

Triple Spiral Press
Sudbury, Massachusetts

Notice
This book and its contents are intended for informational and educational purposes only. It is not a substitute for professional medical advice, diagnosis or treatment. Always consult with your physician or other qualified health professional regarding your medical treatment or with any question you may have regarding a medical condition.

Cover Design and Text Layout: Kate Keleher
Cover Photograph: Jennifer Johnston

Published by Triple Spiral Press
99 Maynard Farm Road
Sudbury, Massachusetts

Printed by AdiBooks
Lowell, Massachusetts

For more information about this book:
www.defeatCFS.net, or e-mail: info@defeatCFS.net

To contact the author: Martha@defeatCFS.net

ISBN: 0-9794769-3-3
EAN: 978-0-9794769-3-8

Printed in the United States of America

Dedication

To John Voyta

I am positive, beyond any doubt, that I never would have gotten well without the unquestioning daily support of my advocate – my husband, John. As I struggled with the cruelty of CFS, he held down a full-time job, took care of an infant and a toddler, did the cooking, grocery shopping, laundry, cleaning and every 2 AM feeding. His willingness to help me track my daily patterns and to develop this protocol through trial and error was unfaltering. When I was at my lowest moments, he reminded me of who I was and who I was determined to be again. As I wrote this book, he was enthusiastic and encouraging. I am blessed to have him as my partner. He has my love and gratitude.

ACKNOWLEDGMENTS

I have been fortunate in my life to be surrounded by wise women and men. Not because they have a lot of college degrees to hang off their names, but because they walk through life learning and growing everyday. They are open to adventure and new perspectives around each bend in life, and their spark of creativity is infectious. They are, with every breath they take, seekers of knowledge who aren't afraid to question or concur with the status quo. For me, it has been a fertile ground to sow my own self-awareness and to seek my own direction. And by example, they have taught me how to handle all that life can throw at you, including my struggle with Chronic Fatigue Syndrome. I am grateful for the gift of their presence in my life.

During my struggle with CFS, the support which I received from my family and friends, my fellow employees and my community, was unwavering and fundamental to my successful return to full health. I especially want to express my love and gratitude to my husband, John, my children, Greg and Carolyn, my mom, Martha, my mother-in-law, Rita, my sisters and brothers, Elizabeth, Stephen, Sean, Jane and Cathy and, finally, my heartfelt gratitude to my friend and emergency go-to woman, Ginny Travers.

For several years I have talked about and worked on this book. Many wonderful and creative friends have listened, encouraged, reviewed and thrown their thoughts into the mix. My thanks to my energizing women's circle, my awesome walking friends, my book group, and especially to my friends Kate Gallion, M.L.S., Lizi Brown, SMFA, Patricia O'Connell, R.N.,

M.Ed., Christine Iskandar, M.S., Lisa Weiss, Ed.M., and Margaret Stewart, M.S.

I want to thank everyone who gave their time and thorough attention to review my manuscript. It is much improved for all their efforts: John Voyta, Ph.D., my husband and biochemist, Sean Kilcoyne, multi-media artist, Deirdre Menoyo, J.D., who also had CFS and is now fully recovered, Vilma Falck, Ph.D., my graduate school professor and mentor, Channing Wagg, M.B.A., writer, David Via, Ph.D., biochemist, Elizabeth Torres, M.D., Diplomate of the American Board of Internal Medicine, Mary McMaster, R.N., and Joel K. Levy, Ph.D., clinical neuropsychologist.

When I "finished" my manuscript, it was just a pile of word documents. I want to thank Kate Kelleher, graphic designer extraordinaire, for her creativity and expertise in packaging my words into a beautiful book. It was my pleasure to work with her.

And many thanks to Jennifer Johnston, fine art photographer, who patiently handled my 2-D phobia and photographed the real me for the book cover.

My thanks to the caring, medical practitioners who helped me during my struggle with CFS. Thank you for practicing medicine "outside of the box".

And finally, thank you to Kira Moore, who was my catalyst for writing this book. I fervently hope that my protocol helps you and others who suffer from Chronic Fatigue Syndrome.

— Martha Kilcoyne

TABLE OF CONTENTS

WHY WRITE THIS BOOK?

In February of 1993 when I was three months pregnant with my second child, I caught a flu virus that permanently changed my life. I lived in the clutches of Chronic Fatigue Syndrome for the next four years struggling to understand what was wrong with me. It shut down my life as I knew it and forced me to become a recluse spending most of my time in bed between short lived efforts to have a "normal" life.

When I started to break free from it, I was subject to relapses. Then there came a time when only thin tentacles of CFS would occasionally reach out to grab me and I would practice the avoidance patterns that I had learned through trial and error, which helped me escape being caught again. Finally, I felt fully healthy once more and blessed to be free of CFS. My reaction to my restored health was instinctive. I ran screaming from CFS as fast and as far as I possibly could. I never looked back. I never talked about it. I tried to never think about it. But the fear that CFS could once again make me bedridden, was imbedded in my subconscious. It was the "deep in your gut" kind of fear that other people have about snakes or "going under the knife." In a corner of my mind, the shadow of CFS still loomed over me, waiting to pounce if I relaxed my vigilance. A few years slipped by without a recurrence.

Then I realized that I needed a way to definitely prove to myself that I was free of CFS and back to normal. My husband and I decided to return to a recreational love that we shared before kids. We signed on to train for and attempt to summit Mount Kilimanjaro in Tanzania, Africa. Everyone, especially my family, thought we were nuts. The people who knew me and who had seen how sick I had been, feared that our crazy plan would only succeed in chaining me to a bed again. We proved them wrong. My triumph over CFS was complete in August of 2000 when I stood in the bright early morning rays of sun on the summit of Kilimanjaro.

Several more years slipped by. The healthy baby girl who was born from that nightmare pregnancy celebrated her 10th birthday. I was home free.

Then one day, I spoke with a friend who had just returned from a trip to visit someone who was ill. When I asked what the illness was, she responded, "Chronic Fatigue Syndrome". I replied, "Been there. Done that." She looked at me quizzically then said, "Oh yeah, I forgot that you had been sick." This brought a smile to my psyche. I had met this friend after my illness and she had only known me as a healthy person. It was hard for her to picture me as sick as her friend. Nothing like tangible evidence of wellness to reinforce your healthful self image and your freedom from disease!

I offered to talk to her friend about the techniques that we had come up with that had been successful for me in the hope that it might help her as well. When I spoke with her friend, I realized that she had come down with CFS at the same time that I had. She had been struggling with CFS for *ten years*!!! I had been completely free of CFS for six years. This rocked me!!

I could only imagine how defeated I would feel if I was still sick. Immediately I asked a barrage of questions and she was pleased to have the opportunity to speak with someone who knew exactly how she felt. The end result was a shock. The protocol that we had come up with that enabled me to get permanently well was not known to her. She had tried some aspects of the protocol, here and there, but not comprehensively and not consistently.

At that moment, in the middle of our conversation, I realized that even though I was free of CFS, I still carried a tiny fearful voice around inside of me. But by the end of our talk, that voice had been silenced. My last vestiges of fear had melted quickly away like a hail stone in the summer heat. I stopped ignoring CFS and finally turned to face it for the first time in ten years. It no longer had the frightening body of a tentacled monster. It couldn't hurt me anymore.

I went straight to the literature and the web. I wanted to know what the state-of-the-art was for CFS ten years later. My findings were disappointing. Although CFS was now a household term, it was still shrouded in mystery. My protocol, or something like it, was scattered about in pieces but wasn't succinctly written up anywhere. And there was still a sizable population of physicians who considered CFS to be a mental illness not a physical one. This seemed unbelievable.

The books that had been written for the lay audience of CFS sufferers were prolific! Some of these books were written by well intentioned practitioners who were missing an understanding of what it was like to suffer from CFS – and subsequently a real knowledge of the *daily* nature of the disease. They focused on long-winded histories of the illness, biological analysis and endless possibilities for treatment. But they missed the point that when you suffer from CFS, you don't have the concentration to add up a column of numbers let alone plow through academic reviews and endless options. A few practitioners who wrote about CFS actually had the disease. They offered some pragmatic advice about many possible medications, alternative medical treatments and hope, but their recommendations still lacked the streamlined simplicity that a CFS sufferer needed. A few authors offered step-by-step programs or protocols but none were a match for the protocol that we had developed. Some books were filled with "ways to stay psychologically healthy." Other books were written by CFS patients who suggested ways to "live with CFS" and cope with managing a near normal life – which was never an acceptable option for me.

Which brings me back to the question I posed at the beginning, why write this book? I wrote it because I wanted to share what I had learned about CFS and how I had reclaimed a healthy normal life. And I wanted to provide this information via a clear, concise protocol written with "brain fog" CFS sufferers in mind. It's one way for me to express the gratitude I have for being well again and, at the same time, to help other CFS patients. Writing this book also satisfied the little part of me that is ticked off that so many people have had to suffer so long without widespread recognition and support.

I'm confident that this protocol will help many CFS sufferers and I am hopeful that for some, it may offer a way to defeat Chronic Fatigue Syndrome and return to a normal life just as I have!

One final note – I am not a health professional nor do I claim to be one. You should consult your physician before starting any course of treatment or changing your medications. My credentials for writing this book are solely based on my experience as a patient suffering from CFS and my trial-and-error (so many errors!) success in returning to normal health. I do have a master's degree in Public Health which provided me with the skills necessary to better understand CFS once I was well, but certainly not when I was sick. My husband has a PhD in biochemistry and was actively researching CFS while I was sick, which was quite helpful, but none of that information actually got me well. The real asset of our formal education during my illness was confidently knowing that academics can often be wrong and that the scientific method of hypothesize, test and analyze, takes time and patience but eventually pays off.

What Is CFS and Do You Have It?

I f you are reading this, mostly likely you, or someone you care about, have been diagnosed with Chronic Fatigue Syndrome (CFS) – also known as Chronic Fatigue and Immune Dysfunction Syndrome (CFIDS). Some researchers also consider Fibromyalgia (FM), Myalgic Encephalomyelitis (ME) and Multiple Chemical Sensitivity (MCS) to be parallel diseases and possibly the same.

CDC Definition

According to the Centers for Disease Control and Prevention (CDC), CFS is "a debilitating and complex disorder characterized by profound fatigue that is not improved by bed rest and that may be worsened by physical or mental activity. Persons with CFS most often function at a substantially lower level of activity than they were capable of before the onset of illness. In addition to these key defining characteristics, patients report various non-specific symptoms, including:

- Weakness
- Muscle Pain
- Impaired Memory and/or Mental Concentration
- Insomnia
- Post–exertion Fatigue lasting more than 24 hours"

Also a patient might experience "sore throat, tender lymph nodes, multi-joint pain (without swelling or redness), or headaches of a new type, pattern or severity."

The CDC states, "The cause or causes of CFS have not been identified."

So you, or your loved one, unfortunately may be suffering from *Chronic Fatigue Syndrome* which has **no known cause** and, as of this writing, **no definitive tests to confirm it**.

CFS is known as a 'wastebasket' diagnosis. Essentially, this means that when presenting a combination of the above symptoms to a Western trained physician, s/he will take your medical history and then methodically proceed to run you through a series of definitive tests to check for possible diagnoses. It is *important*, although exhausting, to go through this process in order to eliminate diseases which have similar symptoms (the majority of which are treatable) such as:

- Mononucleosis
- Autoimmune Disorders (including Lupis, Multiple Sclerosis, etc.)
- Thyroid Disorders
- Adrenal Malfunctions
- Hypoglycemia
- Parasitic or Bacterial Infections (including Lyme Disease)
- Candidiasis (Fungal Infection)
- Dietary Allergies
- Hormonal Disorders
- Chemical or Environmental Sensitivities
- Reactions to Medicines

- Sleep Disorders (including sleep apnea)
- Psychiatric Disorders (including depression)

And this is *not* a complete list. Take the time to be thorough. If you think you have CFS, but have not gone through a thorough testing process, you should. It could save you years of frustration.

Finally, if a physician exhausts the list and finds no match in the standard battery of tests, you can get tossed into the "Other" category and/or sometimes the "wastebasket" of Chronic Fatigue Syndrome. And unfortunately, there are some patients labeled with CFS who have been incorrectly diagnosed.

WHO GETS CFS?

The CDC website lists the following as indicators of who is most at risk for CFS:

- CFS occurs four times more frequently in women than in men, although people of either gender can develop the disease.
- The illness occurs most often in people in their 40s and 50s, but people of all ages can get CFS.
- CFS is less common in children than in adults. Studies suggest that CFS is more prevalent in adolescents than in younger children.
- CFS occurs in all ethnic and racial groups, and in countries around the world. Research indicates that CFS is at least as common among African Americans and Hispanics as it is among Caucasians.
- People of all income levels can develop CFS.

- CFS is sometimes seen in members of the same family, but there's no evidence that it's contagious. Instead, there may be a familial or genetic link. Further research is needed to explore this.

So, if CFS is your diagnosis, there is some solace in knowing that you are not alone in your struggle. According to the CDC, "it is estimated that perhaps as many as half a million persons in the United States may have a CFS-like condition."

CFS – A Cruel Disease

The good news about CFS is that it is not terminal. Your prognosis can be good *if* you take the time to understand the complexity of CFS and its cycles. But it will take a focused effort from you to do this. That's why I consider Chronic Fatigue Syndrome to be a cruel disease. True, it won't kill you. But, it is physically debilitating and there is very little support for getting back to full health again. *You* will have to make it happen yourself if you want to get well again.

A case in point – consider AIDS. People were *dying* from the immune-compromising effects of AIDS and it took nearly a decade for our health system to understand that it was an infectious, deadly disease. Clearly the fact that those dying – in the beginning – were drug addicts and homosexuals, made it easy for health professionals to attribute the deaths to other causes like infections (from needles), other STDs, overdoses, strung-out marginal lifestyles, influenza, etc. For CFS, practitioners just see a very tired person who doesn't test positive for any of the known diseases. They conclude, "Go home and get some rest. You're over stressed and burnt out."

Get used to the idea that you have to manage your own recovery. And that your complete recovery may take at least a full year, possibly longer depending on where you start. You are in this for a while and once you accept this, you'll be ready to get well again.

THE ONSET OF CFS

Most likely, you became sick when several things came into play simultaneously. First, you were probably physically drained and still pushing yourself hard – a perfect host for a disease just looking to move in. In my case, I was three months pregnant, single parenting a two year old (my husband was traveling extensively) and I was holding down a full-time stressful tech support job with some night and weekend hours.

Second, your immune system may have been already stressed by fighting off other minor infections, allergies, environmental exposures, chemical sensitivities, etc. For me, it was February in Boston and I had been experiencing the usual colds, coughs and sniffles.

Third, a particularly nasty flu made the rounds in your circle. It was not uncommon for it to take a week for most people to recover. I was down for two full weeks and still struggling. It never went away.

Note – Although my experience with CFS is labeled as "sudden onset" – meaning that it began as a result of an acute infection that can be identified – some CFS sufferers become sick gradually over a longer period of time. Is it the same illness? Many researchers believe that it is. With gradual onset CFS, it's important to work with your doctor to pay attention to and treat any chronic conditions which may have contributed to developing CFS.

Why doesn't *everyone* come down with CFS? That's not known but some researchers believe that there may be a genetic predisposition for CFS (1). Hormonal misalignments (out of normal balance) have also been studied as possible triggers or causes (2).

What causes the symptoms of CFS? Again, much is unknown, but some researchers believe that the symptoms result from the immune system which is triggered into a dysfunctional state. Somehow the immune system perceives a serious infection or "illness" and fights it. Whether this infection is real or a false reading, the immune system is activated to get the foreign invader under control. Several groups report that a measurable degree of cellular immune activation is associated with the severity of reported CFS-related symptoms (3) or that several types of cytokines – associated with immune response – are elevated in CFS patients(3). The problem seems complicated when the immune system apparently never recognizes success – maybe because it's chasing a "shadow" – and continues to work, day after day leading into a pattern of several months or years. Also, many CFS patients report the reactivation of a latent virus – such as mononucleosis. This indicates a dysfunction of humoral immunity (3).

For me, I was first diagnosed with mononucleosis because my Epstein-Barr titer – the standard blood test for "mono" – was through the roof. When I explained that I already had "mono" as a teenager, I was told that you could get "adult mono" a second time. Ultimately, it became clear that the Epstein-Barr latent virus that I had carried since I had initially contracted "mono" was no longer being kept under control by my "on tilt" immune system and that various other unchecked infections were also on the loose.

In addition to the immune system, the biochemical pathways, including the endocrine and nervous systems, may also be a factor in contributing to CFS (4). A systemic problem may arise where communication between different systems in the body can be negatively effected. Information being passed along may be wrong, reversed or inaccurate. Actions taken as a result of this erroneous information may create more confusion and problems. In general, your mind and body are trying to balance out to a normal healthy state, but the communication network appears to be confused or dysfunctional.

This may also explain why there is a wide array of various symptoms among CFS patients in addition to the "core" symptoms. A systemic immune/bio-pathway problem may present itself differently in each patient, depending on prior medical history and contributing genetics.

So everyone else around you who caught the same "flu" recovered and got back to normal but you were left with most of the following:

- Exhaustion that was beyond fatigue, and sleep that didn't refresh you.
- All over muscle ache and joint pain that persisted and often left you stiff and unable to move with weakness beyond understanding. A persistent sore throat that looked normal upon examination.
- "Thick as a brick" brain fog that kept you from hanging two thoughts together and a frequent inability to remember the thread of a conversation.
- That "coming down with the flu" feeling that never went away.
- Sweats and chills that rarely registered on a thermometer.

- Awareness of unusual heart rhythms.
- Frequent dizziness and vertigo.

These are the core symptoms of what I label as "mainstream" Chronic Fatigue Syndrome. Often this cruel disease forces people to completely give up their normal lives. Most people can't hold down a job – at least not full-time. Active sports participation is out. Anything requiring mental agility is a failure. Taking care of kids becomes a physical trial. Driving reflexes are unpredictable. Every ounce of available energy is used to do the mundane maintenance jobs of life – namely showering, eating, minimum functioning. And any semblance of a social life dissolves into long, lonely days that can really get to you.

Add to all of this, the main reason why I call CFS a cruel disease. After several "bad" days when all of the above symptoms seem to be flourishing despite constant rest, you wake up one morning and feel better. You can actually take a shower and eat breakfast without excessive discomfort. You have a phone conversation and keep up your train of thought. A short walk feels good. You try a trip to the grocery store and, although tired, this is the best you've felt in a long time. Your spirits brighten. You're getting better. You try some housework or maybe cook a nice dinner. If you live with a family, they are thrilled for you when they get home and see what you've accomplished knowing what most days are like for you. You end the day completely exhausted but with an optimism that excites you and leads to expectations for what tomorrow will bring.

The next morning, you can't move. Walking to the bathroom is a major effort. CFS is in full bloom and you completely loose your optimism. It's heartless. It's cruel. It's Chronic Fatigue Syndrome. Accept it and decide to defeat it.

So how do you defeat Chronic Fatigue Syndrome? How do you repair a body/mind system-wide malfunction?

Until medical science identifies a root cause and has developed the treatments to directly restore order to our immune system and biochemical pathways, we need to use what is already available.

The key is to trust the millions of years of evolutionary fine tuning that have resulted in the amazingly resilient, inter-dependent human body. We need to provide our bodies with the tools to self-heal and the supporting environment to succeed. In other words, take the best care of yourself that you can, focusing on the aspects of Chronic Fatigue Syndrome that you have some control over.

On the following page is the Protocol that I used to get well again. Each Step is discussed in this book in detail with guidelines as to how to implement it. Now you need to be ready to apply whatever energy you have to getting well. It's time to get organized and get to work.

Note – This book will not present a complete historical and biological review of CFS, as others have already done that well. But if you want to learn more about the history, latest research, current state-of-the-CFS-art and CFS organizations, refer to the

Resources at the back of this book or use the web to connect with the latest on-line sources. The website of the Centers for Disease Control and Prevention is a great place to start. The more you understand about CFS and the more you are connected with others who suffer from it, the better your chances are to defeat Chronic Fatigue Syndrome.

THE PROTOCOL TO DEFEAT CFS

Step One – Understand Your Version of CFS

Step Two – Find a Doctor Who Will Work With You

Step Three – Break the Cycle of Fatigue

Step Four – Build a Support Network

Step Five – Be Sick! Be a Patient!

Step Six – Fuel Your Wellness

Step Seven – Maintain an Optimal Blood Pressure

Step Eight – Manage Your Stages of Recovery

STEP ONE
UNDERSTAND YOUR VERSION OF CFS

If you sat with a group of CFS patients, you would quickly discover the similarities between your symptoms and experiences with CFS and theirs. The most obvious being: the unrelenting, total exhaustion and pain.

But despite the similarities of symptoms that exist with CFS patients, the actual *patterns* of Chronic Fatigue Syndrome can be markedly different from person to person. Because your immune system/bio-pathways are struggling with a different set of prior medical exposures and predispositions, your version of symptoms will somewhat vary in addition to the shared "core" group. So the first step in the protocol is to understand the unique patterns that describe your own version of Chronic Fatigue Syndrome. Why? This information will give you the perspective necessary to recognize your unique patterns and to track the effectiveness of different strategies.

How? The way to understand your version of CFS is easy. Start keeping a daily record of your symptoms, medications and activities.

The only way I finally saw the negative patterns and was able to break them was via my daily record. Your mind is not sharp with CFS and it can play memory games. The days and weeks melt into an indistinguishable mass and you can't accurately recall the details of the last few days, let alone the past month or two. One of the keys that enabled me to defeat CFS was to break the cyclical patterns, unique to me, that supported the disease. You can find your patterns by keeping a daily record.

DAILY RECORD

So, OK, I'll admit it. The first person who suggested that I keep a daily record was rewarded for their caring with a frown and an audible groan from me. I hated the idea. I was already struggling with daily chores. Another one was not going to help. I was wrong.

Your daily record doesn't have to be long and detailed. It should only take a few minutes to record one day's activity and overall symptoms – a total of 24 hours per entry. As you might have guessed, my record was the briefest possible and yet, it turned out to be one of the important keys for me. I used a simple 81/2 X 11 pad of lined paper and just kept flipping over pages as necessary. I started a new pad when the pages ran out. Use whatever recording method works best for you. For those who like to digitize, a simple word document with running date entries or a spreadsheet would also work well.

The most important information to record:
- Today's date and the time of each entry
- Number of hours you slept the night before
- Medications you took – dosages and times
- Your activities
- Naps and resting periods

- Overall rating of how you felt
- The severity of any specific symptoms that you are tracking

Here is a sample from my frequently minimalist record:

Oct 14   Slept 10-7am   10mg Elavil   75mg Voltarin – twice

              Ate and helped get kids out door

              8-10 rested

              10-12 slept

              12 ate

              1-3 rested

              3-4 did some straightening

              4-6 rested

              6-7 kids and supper

              Rested – everyone to bed

To the right of each day's entry, I noted how I felt overall. This particular entry was: Very stiff muscles and joints, achy and painful, very tired, eyes bothering me, trouble reading.

For me, that entry was a full length novel. Sometimes my notes were shorter for the day's activities. I often wrote "good" or "bad" day for overall symptoms. No symptom entry meant an average day.

The above entry was one of the first I made when I started keeping a daily record. It was shortly after I had a complete relapse in my attempt to return to a normal pace – I had already been sick for a year and a half. That is when I finally realized that if I didn't get serious about managing my recovery, CFS might actually win.

So if you're hoping to defeat CFS, please learn from my mistakes. Keep a daily record and if you miss a day, make an entry for two days the next day. You will be doing this for *at least six months*, most likely longer. So get used to it. It will pay off.

PATTERNS

After you've been keeping your record for a while, you'll begin to see patterns emerge between the quality of your sleep, activity level, good and bad days, type of symptoms and severity, and most important **how much activity you can handle without having to pay for it with a severe set-back.** Getting well from CFS is measured in months and years *not* days. You need to develop a pattern of steady progress forward and avoid the one step forward, two steps back slippage. Think of your recovery as a personal version of the tortoise and the hare race. If you act like the hare, you won't get well. You'll bounce back and forth between feeling better and relapsing. And as I learned, if you let this pattern persist, you risk allowing CFS to get an even stronger grip on you. Steady progress like the tortoise may win back your health permanently.

Other patterns will also emerge from your daily record as you progress toward recovery. At the end of each month:

- Look back over the prior month and find the longest stretches of time that you felt stronger. Study the patterns that preceded this and repeat them.

- Look at specific symptoms and how you tried to address them. What was successful? What was not?
- Don't be quick to pass on something just because you didn't get the result you wanted right away. Keep it up for a longer period of time before you decide if it was or wasn't helpful.
- Look over your activities and rank them according to difficulty or how much energy is required. What can you do easily without a set-back? What is clearly too much for you to handle at this time?
- Are there any combinations of activities that place undue stress on you? Can they be broken up? Spread out?

Sift through your Daily Record for the patterns that will accurately describe your version of CFS and educate yourself. Use this information to adjust your daily schedule and activities.

Long Term Benefit

The ultimate benefit of keeping a daily record is seeing your progress over the long term. This helped me immensely to keep my spirits up when I was frustrated by the snail's pace recovery. Whenever I felt that I wasn't making any progress, I would look back at my entries, four to six months prior, and quickly realize that I was developing a clear understanding of my version of CFS. I could see that I was actually getting healthier and it helped me to recognize that I was definitely moving steadily toward defeating Chronic Fatigue Syndrome.

Step Two
Find a Doctor Who will Work with You

I t's important to build a team of people who will support you through the long process of working toward defeating Chronic Fatigue Syndrome. An important member of your team is a medical doctor. Why? Most importantly, you should work with a practitioner who can help you manage your treatment plan, adjust it appropriately over time and monitor your health. You will probably need access to drug prescriptions and ultimately, if you find the right doctor, s/he will help you to keep up-to-date on CFS and the latest research and treatments.

Limitations of the Medical System

If you have the good fortune to have access to the medical system in the United States, which is the *best* in the western world – my personal bias – then you also know as a CFS patient that getting that same system to focus on an unrecognized illness is beyond frustrating, at times, it can be infuriating.

Western medicine has made giant leaps in the understanding and treatment of disease in our lifetime. And we benefit daily from that expertise. I have a great deal of respect for the quality of our medical schools, our research hospitals and the dedication of our research scientists and clinical practitioners. Our medical schools train young doctors in every known disease and diagnostic method ad nauseam. They know an illness when they are presented with its symptoms. This is a great approach until you have something that is not in a textbook or something which has no test to confirm it. Unfortunately, some doctors have not been given the skill set, perspective or opportunity to look beyond "cookbook" medicine and actually explore the "practice" of medicine.

Then doctors are dumped into the Managed Care System which constrains the available time for, and limits the practice of, "hands on" medicine. Patients with an unrecognized illness are well outside of the normal treatment timeframes when doctors are required to see many patients a day. It must be a blur of faces by the time they leave the office. Primary care physicians do have the luxury of a long-term relationship with many of their patients, but even they have to reread the medical record before picking up the threads of a follow-up visit. A specialist in any discipline rarely has the opportunity to establish a long-term patient relationship.

The good news is that there are many doctors in the system who believe that CFS patients have a physical disease and who will work with you. The bad news is that you may have to sift through a few doctors before you find one.

Here's what happened to me.

After about eight months of being tested and treated by two successive primary care physicians, I was finally referred to an Infectious Disease Clinic at a research hospital. This referral happened because on a scheduled visit to my doctor, I was, for once, presenting the full blown CFS syndrome – fevers to chills, brain fog, full body ache, pain in my joints and total fatigue. When I explained that this was what I'd been trying to describe to her for the last four months, she called the clinic herself and got me an appointment. By this time, she had already tested me for every possible known disease. I was ecstatic. Now I would get the opportunity to be treated by a doctor who might have a clue as to what was happening to me – at this point, I certainly had no idea how to get well. My optimism was – initially – unwarranted.

I was assigned to a doctor who took a thorough medical history, looked over the pages of test results that my primary care physician had sent and gave me a complete physical examination. He explained that he saw nothing remarkable and asked me to keep a record of how I was feeling and return for a follow-up in several weeks. I went home disappointed but returned for the next visit. After he looked over my daily record and briefly examined me, he pronounced his diagnosis.

If you knew me well, you would know that I rarely quote exactly what someone has said to me. I usually couch my recollections of conversations with a disclaimer. I only bet on sure things – hence I rarely bet – and I never play the lottery – unless it's a free play.

However, I quote here exactly what he said because it is forever burned into the cells of my gray matter. He made eye contact with me, straightened his crisp white coat and slowly, in the most caring way that he could muster, he said, "There is nothing physically wrong with you. Go home and have hope, and you'll feel better."

As each one of these words exited his mouth and traveled the five feet to reach my ears, I felt something begin to rise up inside me. It came from the center of my being. From the person who desperately wanted to be well again. From the person who wanted her life back. From the person who was sick of getting no answers. From the person who knew she had a physical illness. From the person who refused to be labeled as a mental case. From the person who wasn't going to take any more unhelpful "bull" from the medical system.

I'm not sure of the exact words that rose up and erupted from my mouth at that moment but it was pure me and unfiltered. With the little strength I had left, I struggled up out of the chair and bellowed something like this, "I am *not* sick because I'm depressed. I'm depressed *because* I'm sick. I was told to come here because this clinic has doctors who know how to treat Chronic Fatigue Syndrome. If you don't know how to treat me, then go out there and find me a doctor who does!" I raised my arm and pointed emphatically toward the door.

His face was flushed red and his hair a bit singed from the heat of my words. He mumbled something and disappeared from the examining room. As I look back on it now, it was my finest manifested vanishing spell.

I fell back into the chair exhausted, totally spent from the effort. I felt bad for the young doctor, but only for a millisecond. It actually felt good to release that frustration. But he didn't come back for a long time. I was starting to think that he might not be coming back at all, and was about to open the door and peek out into the hall when the doorknob turned, and he reentered the room.

He was accompanied by a short balding gray-haired doctor in a wrinkled coat who extended his hand and introduced himself. My heart smiled when he said, "We don't know exactly what's wrong with patients like you, but I've had some success with a few patients and maybe I can help you." Here was a doctor who not only admitted that he didn't know something but was also willing to practice medicine. It was like finding the Holy Grail!

I worked with that doctor for the next year as I slowly climbed out of the CFS hole. Most importantly, he was able to prescribe medications for me that he had used successfully with other CFS patients and he had a knowledge of which drugs were not usually addictive – there will be more about the specific drugs I used in Step Three. He was also an important partner in decision making as I progressed slowly back to health. This was another important key to my successful defeat of Chronic Fatigue Syndrome.

OPTIMIZE YOUR SEARCH

So where do you look for a doctor? Hopefully, ten years after my experience, you won't have to search as long as I did. Try these strategies for optimizing your search:

- Your primary care physician might be knowledgeable about CFS or may know a doctor who treats CFS. If not, your doctor might want to get educated and help you especially if you have a history as his/her patient. It could be a wonderful asset as you work toward recovery.
- If there is a research hospital or medical school nearby, ask about CFS and any members of their staff who are knowledgeable about CFS. Find out if there is a clinic that already sees CFS patients.
- CFS support groups are a great way to network and exchange information about local doctors. Check with the

national CFIDS association (Chronic Fatigue and Immune Dysfunction Syndrome) for local chapters.

- Chat rooms on the internet can be a source for doctor referrals.
- Network, network, network. Talk with everyone you know who has a connection to CFS – another CFS patient, friends, co-workers, relatives and members of your community and religious groups.

When you have a few possibilities, call each doctor's office and speak with the medical assistant at the office – usually a nurse or a physician's assistant. Ask if the doctor is familiar with CFS or treats other patients with CFS. Find out as much as you can before you schedule an appointment or you may be wasting your time and the doctor's. Check with your primary care physician for a referral and check to be sure that your insurance covers visits to this doctor.

Once you've met the doctor, do you feel comfortable with him/her? Does this doctor listen? Do you think that you can work with this doctor? If not, keep looking. Do not waste your time and precious energy trying to convince a doctor that you have a physical illness or trying to make it work if it doesn't feel right. It's *not* worth the effort. When you do find a doctor that's a good fit, great!

WORKING WITH YOUR DOCTOR

Once you have the right doctor, you need to maximize his/her ability to help you. How? Recognize that, most often, when physicians diagnose patients, they are able to treat the cause of the illness. As of this writing, Chronic Fatigue Syndrome is not as well defined or as easily diagnosed, its causes are unknown, and physicians are limited, for the most part, to treating the symptoms. One can only imagine that this must make a caring practitioner feel a little helpless.

So, give your doctor as much information as you possibly can, and be as thorough with your input as you want the doctor to be when considering the best methods for treating you.

Initially, be sure to supply your doctor with:
- A complete medical history
- A complete description of the onset and progression of your CFS symptoms
- The results of all tests that were done by prior physicians – these can be forwarded by the other doctors or your `primary care physician.
- Your daily record
- Medications that you are taking or have taken and your response to them
- The effects of CFS on your life, lifestyle, ability to function, and work

Your new doctor may want to explore a few more possibilities before proceeding with a diagnosis of CFS or even repeat some prior tests. Be appreciative of his/her thoroughness. If CFS is your final diagnosis, continue to supply your doctor with information.

At each office visit:
- Bring your daily record

- Bring your advocate or a member of your support group, if possible
- Describe your symptoms as completely as possible
- Prioritize the symptoms that give you the most discomfort
- Discuss your medications and dosage – prescription and non-prescription
- Discuss any side effects that you may be experiencing
- Discuss your over-all treatment plan
- Listen carefully
- Ask questions about new CFS information

In general, help your doctor to focus on the most critical problems that you are experiencing. Review your medications and whether the doses seem appropriate. Most physicians will start you on low doses and slowly increase them as they determine that you are tolerating the medications without significant side effects. Be patient through this process. Limit the total number of medications that you take. As much as you don't want to be over-medicated, your doctor wants to avoid that situation too.

Decide upon a regular appointment schedule with your doctor and plan the best method for communication when you have a question or problem – phone, fax, e-mail, etc. And remember that your doctor wants you to get well almost as much as you do!

Finding a doctor who will work with you is another important piece in the CFS puzzle. When you find one, you've gotten over a huge hurdle as you work toward defeating Chronic Fatigue Syndrome.

STEP THREE
BREAK THE CYCLE OF FATIGUE

The main symptom that unites all CFS patients, and which ultimately is the reason why they are lumped together in the "wastebasket" of Chronic Fatigue Syndrome is – of course – fatigue.

But this is *not* the kind of fatigue that healthy people complain about at the end of a long day. This is *not* the kind of fatigue that you feel after exerting yourself physically for many hours. This is *not* the kind of fatigue that comes after completing a huge project which drained your brain for several days, weeks or months. This is *not* the kind of fatigue that most people feel post Holiday season. This is *not* the kind of fatigue that makes you fall asleep on the couch at 7 PM at night. This is *not* the kind of fatigue that knocks you down for a week of the flu.

This fatigue is so intense that when it is in full force, you cannot lift your arm above your shoulder and hold it there. You cannot raise yourself out of a chair and walk across a room without collapsing in another chair. You cannot focus your eyes for any extended period of time on printing without strain, blurriness, headache and exhaustion. You cannot hold up a large glass full of water without fearing that you'll drop it. You cannot keep the thread of a conversation. You cannot stand for any period of time. You cannot take a shower without a seat. The bottom line is that you cannot function like an ordinary person who is tired.

Your exhaustion pervades your entire body and it is the foundation upon which CFS builds its hold on you. You must break this hold if you want to defeat Chronic Fatigue Syndrome.

THE FOUNDATION OF CFS

There are three symptoms which appear to link up to form this foundation and ultimately make it worse:

- Muscle ache and pain which effects every inch of your body. Your throbbing neck and shoulders seem to anchor the team of foggy brain, listless limbs and aching back. At times, you can't tell where the focus of pain is located. It seems to reside in every joint and in every muscle.
- Exhaustion and weakness so complete that you can close your eyes and fall asleep at any time of the day or night.
- Your inability to remain in the same position for very long without triggering pain in aggravated joints and muscles.

When healthy people fall asleep from exhaustion, they rest deeply for long periods of time. Usually they awake more rested and refreshed. This rested, refreshed state eludes CFS patients no matter how much time they spend in bed. One of the tools that we need to give to our struggling CFS bodies is deep, restful, rejuvenating sleep. This is one of the tools that we've always used to self-heal and we shouldn't underestimate its restorative benefit.

So, why *can't* a CFS patient get re-energizing sleep and what do you do about it?

Chronic Fatigue Syndrome patients can spend a long night in bed, ten hours or more – apparently sleeping – but they are awakened frequently during the night by pain from complaining joints and other disruptive symptoms. They must shift and move around until they find a new less-uncomfortable position. But now they are awake enough that they have to wait until the exhaustion trumps the discomfort and then they can fall asleep again. Often they're not even aware that this is happening. And this repetitive waking precludes getting into a normal sleep pattern which includes cyclical stages of REM (Rapid Eye Movement) state and the non-REM state that we all require to fully refresh ourselves.

Sleep is broken up into several stages most of which is NREM or non-REM sleep. The first REM stage occurs about ninety minutes after sleep onset. At this point, REM lasts for about ten minutes. Then a new cycle of NREM starts which ultimately leads to longer and longer periods of REM. The longest REM stage – about an hour – happens just before waking after a full night's sleep (5). Although researchers are not in complete agreement about the order and length of each stage or even which stages ultimately are the most important for sleep that is rejuvenating, they do agree that uninterrupted sleep which cycles through both stages is the key.

SLEEP DEPRIVATION

The pattern for CFS patients of long periods of bed rest punctuated every 1-2 hours by waking, creates a sleep cycle which ultimately results in sleep deprivation. The irony is that CFS patients are getting plenty of bed rest but no relief from the fatigue and, at the same time, are actually making their symptoms worse by adding sleep deprivation on top of the CFS fatigue.

Volumes have been written about the short and long-term effects of sleep deprivation and as with any medical field, much is yet unknown. So while the experts are working out the details, we can safely acknowledge that this cycle of sleep deprivation, stacked on top of your totally fatigued body and compromised immune system, exacerbates your symptoms and, after bed rest, you are left with less than when you started.

Let's break this self perpetuating cycle of exhaustion. We'll use three tools: Drugs, Environment and Demands.

DRUGS

As a preference, I usually avoid over-the-counter and prescription drugs. My perspective is to let my illness and symptoms run their course. That way I'm better informed about their severity, and hopefully better able to recognize the healing process and support its progress back to full health. I approached Chronic Fatigue syndrome the same way, initially. I was certain that this was just a minor bump along the path and that I could get well without inventive chemistry. I was wrong. And I wasted a lot of potential healing time by being resistant to their use.

The debate about prescription medications vs. herbal/natural therapies goes on and on. I find myself usually on the herbal/natural side but I do respect and sometimes rely on prescription medications which are targeted and of short duration. When used wisely and carefully, prescription medications can live up to their reputation as the wonder drugs of Western medicine. In my battle against CFS, I eventually chose a complementary blend of both prescription medications and herbal/natural therapies.

Two standard drugs worked well for me and the more experimental drugs were – at least in my case – ineffectual and loaded with side effects. Work with your doctor and explore the possibilities. But ultimately, you need to follow your own instincts and focus on results, which should be your bottom line. When selecting a drug, you should be concerned with compatibility – lack of side effects – and effectiveness. And since you'll be taking it for a long period of time – a year is average – you'll want to stay with non-addictive medications.

Your primary targets are enabling refreshing sleep and alleviating joint/muscle pain.

Nonsteroidal Anti-inflamatory Drugs – NSAIDS: This group of drugs is non-narcotic and is used to relieve pain and inflammation, and to reduce fevers. NSAIDS have a successful track record in treating CFS patients because they alleviate joint/muscle pain as well as stiffness. They are available over-the-counter in recognizable brand names – naproxen (Aleve, etc), ibuprofen (Advil, Motrin, etc) and others. They are also available as prescription drugs – tramadol hydrochloride (Ultram) and celecoxib (Celebrex) as well as others. For the most part, these drugs are considered safe but they can have side effects and possibly – for some patients – dependency. There are many NSAIDS drugs to choose from, some are generic while others are proprietary under specific brand names. The newest class of

NSAIDS are COX-2 inhibitors and they have been under scrutiny for possible cardiac risks and other negative side effects. As always, do your research before starting any new medication.

My doctor recommended a brand of NSAIDS called Voltaren which had proven effective for some of his other CFS patients. The generic name is diclofenac and it is primarily used to treat arthritis and other musculoskeletal conditions. I started with a dosage of 75mg, twice a day, and gradually increased to three a day. This drug builds up its effectiveness over time and for me was very beneficial. Different NSAIDS have varied effectiveness with different patients, so you may need to try a few before you get the best result.

Low-dose Tricyclic Antidepressants: As soon as my doctor recommended a drug in this category, my spirits sagged. Once again, I was being treated like a "head case." But he was very quick to explain that these have been found to be very effective in improving the quality of sleep for CFS patients, and also have a mild pain relief effect. The dose he recommended was a fraction of what is taken to treat depression. Tricyclic antidepressants are doxepin (Adapin, Sinequan), amitriptyline (Elavil, Etrafon, Limbitrol, Triavil), desipramine (Norpramin), nortriptyline (Pamelor) and others.

My doctor prescribed Elavil starting at a 5mg dose one hour before bedtime. Gradually, I worked up to 15mg without a "hungover" feeling. The normal dose for treating depression is upwards of 75 to 100mg per day. After taking Elavil for a few weeks, I noticed marked improvement in my ability to get restful sleep in combination with the NSAIDS. I didn't experience any side effects and continued to take it for almost a year with great long-term results.

Other Antidepressants: If you are experiencing a pronounced degree of depression, your doctor may also recommend a serotonin reuptake inhibitor which is a relatively new antidepressant. There are numerous drugs names in this category – the most widely recognized is probably fluoxetine (Prozac). At my doctors' urging and against my better instincts, I took Prozac for about a month. For me, the side effects were more evident than the benefits and I discontinued it. But I will say that the brain fog lifted some during that period and I got an opportunity to think clearly. It motivated me to work even harder to find the solution to the CFS puzzle.

There are several other categories of drugs which may or may not apply to your situation. Most of them should have been considered when your doctor ran the full battery of tests during your initial diagnosis. These might include treatment of concurrent infections – antibiotics, anti-viral agents, anti-fungal agents and anti-allergy medications. Alone, they have not been found to be helpful in treating CFS unless other conditions are diagnosed. In my humble opinion, other drugs that target symptoms without having an identified cause – anxiety drugs and stimulants are at the top of this list – are a waste of your money and probably just serve to muddy up an already challenged biochemical pathway.

The combination of a NSAIDS with a low-dose tricyclic anti-depressant will definitely target the specific problem of sleep deprivation and finally begin the process of giving your Immune System the opportunity to self-heal. By providing your body with regenerative deep sleep, you will be moving toward regaining your full health once again. But drugs alone won't get the rejuvenating sleep which your body craves.

ENVIRONMENT

Do you *love* your bed? Is it a cozy nest where you melt into the pillow and drift off happily? Do you look forward to the time of the evening when all the "to dos" are done and you can snuggle in? Having a comfortable bed is essential for getting a good night's sleep. I know this sounds like a mattress commercial, but it is so true. When I was ill with Chronic Fatigue, comfort in bed was no longer considered to be a luxury. It became a requirement.

Make sure that your mattress is not too hard and not too soft – one that Goldilocks could love. Experiment with pillows until you get just the right fit. Try a foam shaped pillow if you are having pain and stiffness in your neck and shoulders. Some people get great support from long body pillows. I have always had stiffness in my lower back which became exacerbated to a painful extreme during my illness. A chiropractor suggested sleeping on my side with a pillow between my legs, and it relieved the twisting of my lower back much to my relief. I'm still sleeping that way! Experiment until you feel like you're sleeping on a cloud or as close as you can come.

Evaluate light and noise where you sleep. Get room darkening shades or drape the windows with something so the room is dark to the level that you like. Or try an eye mask. Do everything that you can to ensure that your sleep isn't disrupted by noise. If your noisy environment is not under your control, use correctly fitted ear plugs.

Do you sleep alone? Do you share a bed with a partner? Child? Dog? Cat? Does your partner snore and/or toss and turn?

Does your dog lie on top of you or squeeze you out of bed? Does your child spin and kick at night? Tell them how much you love them but explain how important it is for you to get a good night's sleep – dogs and cats can be trained! Or get a king size bed. Whatever you have to do – make your comfort a priority.

DEMANDS

Just because you are sick, the world and its demands on you don't go away. If you're trying to hold down a job and take care of a family, you're struggling with a load that healthy people can barely manage. You must divest yourself of everything that can go without the earth coming to a standstill. And believe me, many of the things that we do in a day that seem so important, are not critical if they don't get done. More on this in detail later – right now we're focusing on sleep.

You must carve out *ten hours* each and every night that belong solely to sleep. This time must be sacred! Explain this to everyone close to you. People understand if you're straightforward about it. OK, so the dog looks at you blankly when you say you can't get up at 6 AM to let him out to pee. Have someone else in your family take care of the dog for the near future. If you live alone, give a neighbor a key to your place and have them open the door for the dog in the early morning. If you must get up early, go to bed early. Don't go out at night. Just go to bed. *Your social and community activities will still be there when you're well.* Sleep is your highest priority.

Be creative and work it out so that you have your quality sleep. And once you start to see improvement, *Don't Stop!*

Depending on the severity of your struggles with lack of sleep, it will take six months to a year or more to recover from sleep depravation.

Ultimately, breaking the cycle of fatigue is dependent on you getting a full night of restorative sleep of *at least ten hours*. It should be your highest priority if you hope to defeat Chronic Fatigue Syndrome. And as we continue through the protocol and identify other tools to help your body self-heal, quality sleep will be the foundation upon which you work your way back to full health.

STEP FOUR
BUILD A SUPPORT NETWORK

If you want to defeat Chronic Fatigue Syndrome, your chances of doing it without help are slim. Why? Because you need to rest and heal – that has to be your only job. And you won't be able to do that if it seems like your life is falling apart. Personal, financial, professional and social responsibilities will haunt you with guilt. Contrary to what your body is telling you, you'll drag yourself out of bed and try to hold things together. You'll fall into the CFS trap of one step forward and one or more steps back. And the longer you suffer and yo-yo with CFS, the higher the probability will be that you'll set up a recurring pattern that your immune system won't be able to break. I wasted a year and a half yo-yoing until I allowed myself to rest and heal. Please don't repeat my mistake.

The physical and mental challenges of struggling with CFS are debilitating enough. You need help. You need a support network.

RECRUIT A PERSONAL ADVOCATE

Your doctor is an important member of your network. You'll also need a personal advocate. Someone who is your primary support in getting through the day-to-day struggles of recovery and the day-to-day maintenance of living. If you're lucky, you'll have more than one.

What does an advocate do? An advocate takes on several roles.

- Emotional and Moral Support
- Evaluation Support – Provides an Objective Opinion
- Basic Daily Maintenance Support
- Solution Support – Ideas
- Research Support

An advocate is someone who *knows you well.* This person has been in your life for a long time. This person knew you when you were strong and making your life happen. This person understands your personality strengths and flaws. This person sees all your blemishes and *still* loves you. This person is not perfect either and you *still* love her/him. This person knows your patterns of behavior and is certain that you would not indulge yourself in excuses. This person does not need to be convinced that you have a physical illness. This person wants you to be well again as much as you do.

What are you asking this person to do? This person needs to be willing to devote a significant amount of time to your recovery. First, your advocate needs to be willing to listen. And listen some more. This advocate will talk with you every day throughout your illness. This advocate will hold you up emotionally when you don't have the strength to do it yourself. S/he will remind you of who you were and what you can do once again. S/he will make you keep to your plan for breaking the destructive cycles of CFS. And this will not be easy to do given the up-and-down nature of your energy levels and the cruelty of CFS.

Your advocate is also your lifeline to the normal world to which you desperately want to return. S/he will keep you connected to all the other people in your life who you miss but can't muster the energy or time to contact. S/he will know when you most need that phone call from someone or have the strength/need to reach out.

Your advocate is also a sounding board for honest opinions about what activities you're ready to try or when you need to wait a little longer. This perspective is invaluable as you try to see the long view of your illness and where you are on the path to full recovery. Your advocate reinforces the small successes that will finally add up to long-term progress and, conversely, helps you to recognize mistakes that lose you ground. Half the success of avoiding mistakes is recognizing what they are and not repeating them. This may seem elementary but when your thinking is CFS fuzzy, it's hard for you to see patterns that may be obvious to someone else.

Your advocate is the person who will help you with basic daily maintenance and/or with creative solutions to your everyday maintenance and survival while you're recovering. This person will help you recruit a network of people around you to help. And finally, s/he will also help you to keep up with the latest CFS info and research.

And yes, this is *a lot* to ask of someone. But understand that your advocate will feel better helping than feeling helpless while watching you struggle.

Who is this fabulous angel? It could be your spouse, partner, sibling, parent, child, family member, good friend, or close neighbor. Most likely, it's someone with whom you've already been sharing your frustrations with your CFS diagnosis. Although it's wonderful if your advocate lives with you or near by, s/he can be someone you talk to over the phone. Maybe you'll have one close and another at a distance.

I was blessed that my husband, John, was my personal advocate. Although we didn't truly understand the role of an advocate at the time, we began to understand, during the course of my recovery, just how important he was to my successful defeat of CFS.

How do you recruit your advocate? Hopefully, you have identified someone who is already trying to help but may be floundering, unsure of what to do. Call them and talk about your need for someone to be there for you each and every day. Share this book with them as it may help you to articulate your needs. Be clear about the long haul. You need to have this person's full commitment and any reservations might create problems when you need them most. Most likely, you've chosen the right person. And if they're not sure, trust that they're being honest with you, and look for someone else.

What if you can't identify an advocate? You may not be able to find an advocate right away. Your "advocate" may actually be several people who help you as part of your support network. Be open to how "advocacy" will work for you. Your need for objective opinions, reinforcement of your pace, reminders of who you are, coordination of your daily needs, etc., may be met in different ways. You *will* find just the right fit. Be open to how your version of "advocacy" will work.

THE REST OF YOUR SUPPORT NETWORK

In order to completely recover from CFS, you will need to devote all your energy and time to getting well. As you begin to recognize the patterns that perpetuate your illness, you will need to break them. And breaking them will require you to abandon the pace and style of your life – for a while. You will have to make drastic changes in your daily schedule. This will involve a lot of rest. How do you rest and take care of yourself with all the demands of a 21st century lifestyle? It isn't easy. I struggled with this every day.

At the height of my symptoms, I could barely care for myself, let alone the needs of children and family. Some days, just walking across the room crippled me with fatigue. Driving was dangerous because my reflexes were in slow motion. This meant that I couldn't go grocery shopping or run errands, even if I had the energy to do it. I couldn't clean or cook for long. I had about two waking hours a day that were not devoted to eating, dressing/showering or resting. If you go back and read the sample entry for my daily record in Step One, you will understand what I mean.

Depending on your Stage of Recovery – more about this in Step Eight – what you are able to handle on a daily, weekly and monthly basis will vary. And as you recover, you'll be able to progressively do more.

So here's a list of daily energy demands that most healthy people can manage. For someone in the most acute stage of CFS, they become an attempt to climb Mount Everest.

• Personal hygiene – showering, shampooing and dressing.

- Preparing, serving and cleaning up after at least two meals a day
- Basic daily cleaning and straightening
- Child care
- Pet care
- Laundry
- Weekly cleaning – bathrooms, floors, vacuum cleaning
- Bill paying and piles of important paperwork regarding your illness
- Helping with school homework

Now you leave the House:

- Grocery Shopping
- Shopping for other necessities
- Filling Prescriptions
- Driving to appointments – you and other family members
- Getting kids to school (or bus stop) and back
- Driving car pools to activities and back
- Walking the dog

This is just the minimum to keep your life afloat. If most of these things don't get done, you'll suffer. Some of them *can* slide and it won't be tragic. Honestly, my house was a complete dirt bin while I was sick. Sometimes it bothered me but I had to learn to close my eyes and let it go. Decide what is critical and find a way to get it done by someone else. Work with your advocate to identify people who can help you. You've probably already heard, "If there's anything I can do, let me know." OK, realistically, some of those people don't mean it. But most of them were sincere. And the reason why they don't follow up with a phone call is because they're afraid to wake you up. So call them and let them pick up small chunks of your life here and there. It will add up to a huge energy savings for you. And they'll feel good about helping.

As you network, remember to avoid dumping too much on one person for too long. Good will can get strained over the long haul. Your advocate can help you to be aware of how your helpers are holding up. S/he can be a neutral go-between and get the honest answer that you might not. And remember to give your advocate a break now and then too.

INCOME

What about money? You can probably let many things slide but income is a crucial need. I could not work and earn a living during my struggle with CFS. Luckily, I earned only half of the income in my family. Even so, we barely managed to get by. What do you do if you're single or earn the only income in a family? Talk this over with your advocate and your family. Be realistic and straightforward about what you think you can handle in terms of work and what you can't. And be prepared to have to re-evaluate this after you give it a try. Trial and error regarding what you can handle will be a normal CFS recovery pattern – and in *all* aspects of your life – until you get it right. Would part time be a short term solution? Could a non-working spouse contribute for a while? Can you earn income from home? Would moving in with a family member or friend eliminate the demand for a lot of income during your recovery? Think creatively to come up with workable solutions.

Don't forget about health insurance. Fortunately, I qualified for short term disability through my work which eventually turned into long term disability. It wasn't a lot of money and I had to go through an exhausting process – for someone with CFS – to get it and to keep it. But together with my husband's salary, it enabled us to just keep up with our mortgage payments and pay for two kids in childcare. Discuss insurance options with your employer. Be sure to check with the Social Security administration as they also offer disability payments if you qualify. If you are on disability, most likely, regular appointments with your doctor will be required to document your progress, functional capacity and, eventually, your ability to return to work.

Explore all the options that you feel are available. Your goal is to reduce or eliminate your need to work while lowering your need for income to support you and your family. And remember to focus on this being a *temporary* solution. If you cut back and make good progress toward breaking the cycles that perpetuate CFS, in six months to a year, you will probably be able to begin taking on more again. And don't forget the other half of the income equation – spending. Cut your expenses down to the thinnest margin possible. Live cheap. Eat cheap. Be frugal.

CHILD CARE

I was pregnant with my second child when I became sick with CFS. After she was born, I was briefly better, then had a complete relapse. So another area where I struggled was functioning well enough to be responsible for a baby and a toddler. At first, I couldn't handle them at all. I was so weak that I didn't trust myself to pick up and hold my baby daughter. I couldn't stay awake to watch my exploring three year old and certainly couldn't handle keeping him from harm. They were both in full time daycare – a luxury which we scrimped to afford – until my son was five and my daughter was two. By that time, I was well enough to be able to care for them with some limitations. Luckily, my son entered kindergarten starting with an afternoon program. I would put him on the bus and then I would tuck the baby and myself in for a nap. Often, I would wake from a deep sleep to her loud crying on the baby monitor and realize that the alarm had been going off for half an hour. I'd been out for almost three hours. Fortunately, she had an internal clock synchronized with the school bus schedule. Frequently, I was awake just long enough to drag myself to the front door and wave weakly to the bus driver so he would let my son get off.

If you have kids, you will have a huge challenge. Work with your advocate to explore every possibility. You may be lucky enough to have a parent or family member who can help with the kids a couple days a week. Explore bartering with another parent for childcare. Be creative. You're not the only parent struggling with the costs of childcare.

NECESSARY PAPERWORK AND INFORMATION GATHERING

Depending on your situation, you may or may not be capable of dealing with formal matters like health insurance paperwork, bills, networking and general research about the latest CFS information. You'll need to be in contact with insurance representatives and other agents of the "system". You'll want to get answers about CFS – not that you'll find them but that won't keep you from wanting to look. And networking with other CFS patients can be a good boost to your morale. They won't have all the answers either but commiserating can help and you will get tips along the way that pay off for your steady progress back to full health.

Try to give yourself a small window each day to pay a few bills, or make an important phone call, or to connect with information via the internet. It will get something done each day and give you the permission not to lie in bed awake worrying when you should be sleeping. Work with your advocate to come up with a workable schedule.

Once you've set up a means to hold your life together while you're working toward defeating CFS, you'll realize quickly that the stress of being sick is dramatically reduced and the unmet demands of your life aren't nagging at you and keeping you from healing. This reduction in the 'worry factor' and the increase in valuable restorative rest will be appreciated by your immune system as it labors to return to a healthy, normalized level of functioning.

And don't forget to thank your advocate/s everyday which is important in allowing yourself to be a patient as you'll see in Step Five.

Step Five
Be Sick! Be a Patient!

U ltimately, even if you apply yourself whole heartedly to following through with the other steps in this protocol, you will *not* defeat Chronic Fatigue Syndrome unless you allow yourself to be sick and act like a patient. That may sound simple but each of us has a lifetime of learned attitudes that can create obstacles which keep us from accomplishing the obvious.

The realtor's adage of the three most important points when buying real estate, "Location, location, location" is an apt parallel. It doesn't matter if the roof sags, the plumbing leaks and the layout is awkward. All of these things can be fixed or renovated. But if the house is on a highway or floods every spring when the snow melts, there's very little you can do to fix it. The similar CFS adage would be "Attitude, attitude, attitude." The way in which you choose to approach CFS will determine whether you can defeat it or CFS defeats you.

Attitudes

There's been a lot written about classic personality types. Most people know if they're a Type A or a Type B. Some have taken more sophisticated personality tests like the Myers Briggs Type Indicator or the Keirsey Temperament Sorter. Whatever your experience has been, the majority of people have a reasonable clue as to how they approach stressful, frustrating or physically challenging problems. I'm not a psychoanalyst but I've observed that in general CFS patients frequently fall into one of the following categories in response to their illness. See if you can recognize yourself.

What Illness? – These patients are often in *denial* about being sick or the need to follow any type of modified routine. Or even if they recognize their illness, they still choose to push through it – whatever it takes on a daily basis. They drag themselves around day after day, then crash when they absolutely have to. CFS loves patients who do this and has the potential to set up permanent residence. For many CFS sufferers, their body can't keep doing this. This pattern of behavior can eventually set them up to suffer a major relapse.

Half and Half – These patients "get it", but only half of the time. They seesaw back and forth between adjusting their lifestyle in order to get well and jumping back on the Merry-Go-Round the moment they start to feel better, until they fall off again. Up and down, up and down, up and down – where's the sense in this kind of cycle? This pattern of behavior has the potential to set them up for CFS to become deeply ingrained and possibly worse.

Oh, Woe Is Me – After struggling with CFS for a while, these patients accept their misfortune to have contracted

CFS and seem to give in to a permanently "sick" lifestyle. I wouldn't go so far as to say that they act like hypochondriacs, but they allow CFS to control their lives rather than taking proactive steps to control CFS. They don't get any worse but they accept the disability with a depressed resignation. These patients manage to "live" a disabled existence with CFS.

I'm the first to admit that there are many different coping styles, and that a CFS sufferer could potentially follow one of the above scenarios and return to full health, but for me, none of these attitudes would be successful in defeating CFS. I took a turn at "What Illness?" before I dabbled in "Half and Half" for a while. Then I started acting like I "got it" but only long enough to feel measurably better before I slipped back into "Half and Half" again.

With hindsight, I can see that this approach was completely ineffectual for me, not to mention risky. Finally, I "got it" on a full-time basis, thanks to serious pressure from my advocate, my husband, John. He helped me to see, that in my case, I was allowing CFS to set up permanent residence in my body. I learned, the hard way, that I needed to adopt a new perspective – one which accepted CFS as a daily reality and the accompanying *temporary* lifestyle adjustments required by me, to defeat it.

I'm not going to pretend that this attitude adjustment was easy. It pushed me to the limit of what I could admit about myself. I don't recommend illness as a good way to get to "know yourself", but when CFS has taken up residence in your body, you don't have a lot of options. Start taking a careful look at yourself and your attitudes if you plan to defeat CFS.

YOUR PERSPECTIVE

The way that you view your illness and yourself as a sick person can influence how soon you can be well again. At one extreme, we're all familiar with the "Teflon Don" type personality who never sees him/herself as part of the problem or who is never willing to accept responsibility – or the dreaded "blame" – for a failure.

At the other extreme, many of us can be unkindest to ourselves when we are faced with a problem. "It's me. I'm at fault. I brought this on myself. I'm not good enough. If only I was stronger, smarter, quicker, more attractive, more resilient, more resourceful, etc." We tend to be the judgmental type that is more critical of ourselves than others. This self-critique can get to our inner most feelings where we all know how to hurt ourselves the most. If you are suffering from CFS, you have endless fodder for this negative path. And you can do a great deal of damage during the endless idle hours.

Decide not to take this path. Decide to cut yourself some slack. Decide to recognize your lack of control over getting sick. OK, we'll let you have "I shouldn't have been pushing/working so hard" but that's in the past now anyway. Decide to accept your need to "be sick" so that you can get well again. Decide to take control of CFS rather than gnash your teeth over it. Decide to reserve your emotional and psychological energy for productive work, not destructive recrimination. Decide to be kind to your inner self who is "really angry over being sick". Decide to give yourself a "Get Out of Blame Free" card. Decide to let all that negative energy go…

You need to use your energy to build up your determination to defeat CFS. You need your energy to be proactive.

OTHER PEOPLE'S PERSPECTIVE

If it's a struggle to get yourself to lay off the self criticism, you know that it's nearly impossible to get others to give you a break. For all of our "good will" and generous intentions, people are lightning fast to judge others. Pair that with our weakness for making assumptions and we can pigeon hole others in a millisecond. Add CFS into the mix and it seems like people can quickly become condescending. Or are we just assuming that they are thinking the worst?

Our perceptions of how other people view us can get bogged down with many variables. Not to mention all of our *own* assumptions and judgments. Sorting it all out could take years of analysis. And for what? Will other people's perceptions of us really affect our lives?

Have you ever heard of the 20-40-60 rule? It's basically that at the age of 20, you are constantly concerned about what other people think of you. By the time you're 40, you begin to realize that you don't really care that much about what others think of you. And finally around 60, it dawns on you that no one was ever that preoccupied with you because they were caught up in their own little spheres of self doubt.

What can you do about what others think of you and your CFS diagnosis? Absolutely nothing. Be magnanimous and cut everyone else some slack while you're cutting yourself some. If people sympathize and can help you in some way – wonderful. If they judge you as a slug and a head case – so be it. Let it go.

Otherwise, you'll just be letting them suck up your energy which you should be guarding as a precious commodity. Lean on your advocate for a truthful assessment of where you are and what you can handle. Use your Support Network to bolster you when you need it.

Decide to let all those other people's opinions go...

Your Behavior

You have many options for how you choose to adjust to having Chronic Fatigue Syndrome. They range from completely self-supportive to totally self-destructive. The actions you take can affect your ability to get well again.

Decide to understand your version of CFS. Decide to find a doctor who will work with you. Decide to break the cycle of fatigue. Decide to build a support network. Decide to allow yourself to be sick, be a patient. Decide to fuel your wellness. Decide to maintain an optimal blood pressure. Decide to manage your stages of recovery. Decide to be well again.

Your behavior is under your control.

Other People's Behavior

Other people's behavior is *not* under your control.

Ignore judgmental remarks. Let rude stares and affected facial expressions pass right through you. Don't dwell on the phone that never rings anymore. Don't let lack of contact with former circles eat at you. Above all, avoid making assumptions about other people's behavior. Many people truly do not understand CFS, just as you didn't before you got sick. Explain what you can and then let it go. You will have plenty of opportunity to pick up the pieces of your former life when you are well again. You may even realize that you're better off without some of those pieces.

Appreciate those who understand and support you. Have gratitude for your support network. Remember to tell your advocate/s how much you love them and value their commitment to getting you well again. Be open to unexpected generosities from others.

Decide to let all the other people's behaviors go…

I'M DEPRESSED *BECAUSE* I'M SICK

When patients, doctors and friends talk about Chronic Fatigue Syndrome, depression is the elephant in the room. After all the tests are run, after all other avenues of diagnosis are exhausted, after the "wastebasket diagnosis" of CFS is pronounced, most providers and support people are thinking depression.

In defense of the medical practitioner, from their perspective, they've done a thorough screening and have not found any evidence of a physical illness. And by the time the seemingly endless process of testing and diagnosis is finished, the patient has a high degree of frustration and disappointment. The patient seems to have a mental illness.

And by this point, what patient wouldn't be feeling let down, discouraged and bordering on depression? Although no one wants to have most of the things that they've been tested for, at least it would be an answer. Something to know, to understand, to come to terms with and to begin to deal with. For most patients, it's the first time in their lives when the medical profession hasn't been able to treat and correct a serious illness they were presenting. So after the CFS diagnosis is delivered, the patient is let down *and* still left with exhaustion, pain, brain fog, all over body aches and debilitating physical symptoms.

Other than the gross assumption by some practitioners that mental illness is the "cause" of CFS, the truly unfair aspect is that initially, the patient doesn't know this. It's one of those dirty little secrets that the "rookie" isn't in on. The patient *knows* that there is something physically wrong with them. They feel it at a system-wide level that can't be easily described. They struggle to find words that can express how awful they feel. I finally came up with an engine metaphor. It felt like I was a four-cylinder engine only firing on two with the timing way off!

For the astute patient, despite the brain fog of CFS, this attitude toward their illness quickly becomes apparent. All treatment comes to a halt. They are sent home with doctor's orders to rest and get out for some walks. As one of my doctor's dared to say to me, "Go home and have hope and you'll feel better." Patients are often prescribed anti-depressant medication or, at least, there is an initial conversation about it. Believe me, this *really* cheers the patient up.

So now the CFS patient begins down the path of questioning. Everything is up for reconsideration. But they are still left with this physically debilitating disease that now is the patient's "fault". When the medical professional says, "We can't find anything *physically* wrong with you," how do they expect the patient to take it?

For me, I was deeply discouraged and went home with no answers and a broken spirit. Throw in a few months of isolated bed rest and you have a fertile host for depression.

Prior to CFS, I wasn't a person who was subject to struggles with depression. I had my "blue" days every so often but I'm basically an optimist and didn't stay down for long when I was feeling low. CFS was my first experience with physical and mental discouragement that didn't go away. It took a long time for me to recognize it for what it was and then to name it as a side effect of my illness *but not the cause of it.* My response to those who named my illness as depression was, "I'm *not* sick because I'm depressed, I'm depressed *because* I'm sick!"

I freely admit that I made many mistakes trying to understand my emotions during the course of my CFS years. Dealing with depression was overwhelming for me. Add in my "Super Woman Feminist" streak which is a wonderful asset when wielded as a tool but an unforgiving weapon when self-inflicted. Even after I "got it" and started allowing myself to act like a patient, there were many long hours/days/weeks/months of doing what I was supposed to do and hating it.

During my first "Half and Half" phase, I made two disastrous attempts at returning to work in a half-time capacity. I was four months pregnant and then five months pregnant during the two successive attempts at normalcy. These misguided efforts resulted in a total relapse. At the time my diagnosis was still "adult mono" with the prognosis that I would not be able to recover until after I gave birth.

So, I lay exhausted in bed, hour after hour, day after day, week after week, staring at the calendar on the wall through a thick brain fog. With each passing day my belly grew larger and larger, and I struggled to get into comfortable positions despite my joint and muscle pain. My condition was not improving. All the bed rest possible wasn't getting me well because of the pregnancy. Exhaustion was a permanent companion. Time was slipping through my fingers and I let the frustration gnaw at me.

I worried about never getting well again. I worried about the baby and if she would be OK given how sick I was. I worried about all the things I wasn't doing to support my family. I worried about how exhausted my husband was, taking on everything. I worried about my three year-old son and how I wasn't mothering him. I worried about our home which had degraded into a dirty pit. I worried about the rest of my family and how out of touch I was. I worried about my sister-in-law who was seriously ill with cancer. I worried about her family and what I wanted to be doing for them. I churned things over and over and over. I allowed what little energy I had to be sucked up needlessly and squandered. Yes, all of it was important. But I wouldn't allow myself to accept my situation and to use my precious energy intelligently. Instead, I decided to squander it on guilt. Little did I know that, comparatively, this part of my illness was easy. The worst was still at least a year into my future.

Finally, the calendar was flipped over and there, blessedly, was a large X boldly marked with black felt tip marker on July 28th. My obstetrician had scheduled me to be induced into labor that day so that the birth was under the best possible circumstances given my inability to handle a drawn-out labor. When that day finally came, it was a wild and scary ride for me. I give my obstetrician a lot of credit for getting me through it. And it resulted in the birth of a healthy girl – Sumo-sized. It was a relief to know that all my energy had been drained in order to nurture her. Once again, my faith in the cycles and interdependencies of nature was validated.

And within a week I was feeling stronger and healthier than I had for five months. My spirits soared as I looked toward reestablishing my old life, returning to work and being able to contribute to my family once again. Unfortunately, this did not happen.

Although the diagnosis of "adult mono" was a complete fiction, the prognosis had been correct. I wouldn't get well until after I delivered the baby. But my quick bounce back after the baby was born, was short lived. Even before I went back to work, I knew that something was still physically wrong with my system. My wellness was becoming a physical and emotional game of "Chutes and Ladders". Every ladder gave me strength and hope, and every chute dumped me back even further.

It took only a few months of attempting to return to work before I had a complete relapse. Ultimately, the final chute that I allowed myself to slide down dumped me off the board and out of the game. I landed lower than start, worse off than I had ever been in the entire course of my illness. Not only was I a physical wreck with exhaustion, pain, stiffness and brain fog, I crashed with a loud thud on the cement floor of my emotional psyche. When I dragged myself upright and peered around, I was in a dark, unfamiliar space. My state of mind at this point was fragile. I felt so defeated by this nameless thing that had invaded and derailed my body.

At this time, as I've described in Step Two of the Protocol, I was seeing a new primary care physician. She was sympathetic but also uncertain as to the cause of my illness. She methodically put me through the correct process of ruling out all the possible medical causes of my presenting symptoms and, for her efforts, I will always be thankful.

Unfortunately, when she had exhausted all possible paths, even she began to see me as a long-term postpartum depression patient – *which I wasn't*. Fortunately, she also still had a physician's intuition that something else was not right. When she referred me to the Infectious Disease Clinic at a local teaching hospital – even though I had to fight to get to the right doctor – this was the beginning of my true recovery. It had been *a year and a half* since I had first come down with CFS. But there was one more, dark place I had to visit before I left behind the depression that was a side effect of CFS.

Shortly after the rookie doctor gave me the "Go home and have hope" speech, I was *so* frustrated with my roller coaster days that I decided that maybe he was right. It might just *be* a head game. I determined to live a normal life and to push through the pain and exhaustion. My husband, John, shook his head and said that I was setting myself up for a relapse but I didn't listen. I had yet to fully understand the role of an advocate.

So the next day, I rose and threw myself stubbornly into my life. Although I was not working at the time because I had lost my job due to my illness, I cleaned the house, ran errands, shopped for groceries and cooked dinner. By the end of the day I was physically spent but mentally high. It felt wonderful – positively ecstatic - to have a chunk of my life back. Day two was difficult, but I took pain killers and pushed myself to add exercising into another active, physically demanding day. Day three was a struggle to get out of bed but I was certain that this was the break point that I had to surpass. It could be the key to defeating CFS. Looking back, that decision would definitely make my "Top Ten Worst Decisions of My Life" list. I took my pain killers and literally willed my exhausted body to carry itself through the day. By the afternoon, my exhaustion, pain and fog became so extreme that I imploded and collapsed into bed.

As I lay in that fetal stupor, feeling acute pain and not having the strength to even move my hand, I knew that my battery had been completely discharged. I was totally empty - devoid of any source of energy other than the pervasive, screeching pain. Only my brain showed a faint sign of self awareness. It was silently chanting a self-incriminating mantra, "Stupid…stupid… stupid…stupid…" When I was at the lowest point of my illness, I chose to kick myself a little more. Not a recommendation made by any credible self-help guide. John was mercifully gentle and said simply, "I hope you've gotten *that* idea out of your system now."

It was the worst day of my illness. There was only one positive thing I could take from it – a giant leap forward on the CFS learning curve. Although I always knew that CFS was a real physical illness, now I had tangible self-validation. And the true head game of CFS was not fighting off the deep frustration that accompanied it, but instead it was taking control of CFS and proactively working toward getting well again.

Decide to pour your limited energy into the positive head game of regaining your wellness and let that negative, self recriminating head game go…

TECHNIQUES FOR HANDLING THE HEAD GAME

Three approaches work well when struggling with the CFS head game.

Stay Connected – The resting and recovery routine for CFS can be inherently isolating. Use several strategies to stay connected. At least once each day, call someone on the phone just to talk or send/read a few e-mails. Or login to an on-line chat room – and it doesn't have to be about CFS, sometimes it's nice to pursue other interests. Or read a blog. Or even create one for your friends who want to keep tabs on how you're doing. If you're able to go out, support groups that are positive can also keep you connected – and you may even find a virtual one. Ask a neighbor or friend to stop in for a cup of tea – with the understanding that your friend prepares the tea, serves the tea, cleans up after the tea and ignores your messy house while you sit and thoroughly enjoy the company – this is a true friend.

Stay Productive – Despite your brain fog and exhaustion, there are a few things you can do each day that contribute to keeping your life on track. Pay a bill or two – on-line banking allows you to queue payments for future dates or just date the envelope for mailing later. If you need to shop for just about anything, you can find it on-line. If shipping charges are prohibitive, set up a relationship with a local store and have a member of your support network pick up your order. Make an insurance or employment related phone call. Schedule a doctor's appointment. Make a grocery list – nowadays you can even order groceries on-line and have them delivered at a cost. Or ask a member of your support group to pick up your order. Surf a little. Check out CFS sites for the latest info or research. Use on-line access to your local library to request books, CDs and Videos – and, of course, have a member of your support network do a weekly library trip for you. Depending on your stage of recovery – more about this in Step Eight - you can be productive on a larger scale. Organize those old photographs into albums, write that short story, take an on-line course for college/graduate credit, do part time work from home, etc.

Stay Relaxed – It's important to intentionally let go of the stress and guilt of being sick. Be mindful of your need to relax and heal with positive energy – not negative recrimination. Find something that works for you or a combination of several. Breath deeply, meditate, visualize yourself healthy, listen to music, stretch – as you are able, use aromatherapy – oils or incense, etc. Avoid cranking through the endless list of things that you are *not* doing. Instead focus on creating ways that you *can contribute* – think "outside of the box." We live in a virtual age where anyone with a computer and access to the internet can make things happen.

ROUTINE, ROUTINE, ROUTINE

During my struggle with CFS, I learned that the best strategy for being a patient, is to be a slave to routine. My most productive reclaiming of health was accomplished during the phase when I affectionately – for the most part – called my advocate "The Jailor".

It was shortly after my disastrous attempt to prove that CFS was not a physical illness but only a head game. By this point, my advocate and husband, John, had sympathetically watched my long roller coaster ride with CFS. He had the vantage point of an observer who could see patterns that were not obvious to me. Certain cycles were starting to look familiar to him and he wanted to try setting up a daily schedule that would reinforce the positive patterns and avoid the negative ones. At first, I found this input welcome and somewhat of a relief. Until I realized how incredibly restrictive it was.

Here was my typical day:

7 AM	Get up and eat breakfast with John and the kids. Wave goodbye when they leave for work and daycare. Straighten up the kitchen. Sit at my desk for a while to try to do some work.
9–11 AM	Nap
11 AM	Get up and take a shower, then dress. This took about an hour to do with periods of rest between each step.
Noon	Eat lunch. Try to read or work at my desk.
2–5 PM	Nap
5 PM	Get up and read or work
6 PM	Eat dinner with the family.
7 PM	Go to bed. Sometimes my four year-old son "read" me a bedtime story before his dad tucked him in.

Imagine doing this for several months! Weekends were a bit different but all the naps still took place. Even though this routine was starting to pay off after one month, John insisted that I not alter the amount of rest. I chafed against this limitation but slowly, after three straight months of monotony, I started to understand that he was onto something.

At the same time, I was finally seeing a doctor who was helping me to break the cycle of fatigue – Step Two of the Protocol – with the appropriate medications to maximize the quality of my sleep and to alleviate the intensity of my pain.

So, I finally embraced "the schedule" and over time, I got stronger, slowly but continuously with no major slip backs. I added in other activities and cut back on the naps over time. And although I was restless to get "back to normal", this was real, *sustained* progress and I understood that my patience would be rewarded with a return to full health. And I relied on my advocate to keep me honest about what I could handle and what I couldn't.

Keep in mind the following:

- Rest – Be a patient and have patience! Nap every day.
- Be on a daily schedule with *short* windows for work, reading, e-mail or making phone calls to stay in touch with friends.
- Only sleep in bed – Don't live there. Get out of bed when you're not napping. Sit in a comfortable chair. Sit outside in the fresh air or in the sunshine.

- Take a shower and dress every day, even if it takes several rest periods to get through it. Being clean and fresh is good for your spirits.

PATIENCE, PATIENCE, PATIENCE

Slow, steady progress is crucial to defeating CFS. Yes, it's a long, potentially boring timeline. But it's *temporary* and the reward may be a complete return to wellness with CFS in your rear view mirror.

So, slow down, physically and mentally. Allow yourself to Be Sick. Allow yourself to be a patient. Set up a daily and a weekly routine that you can handle without backward slippage. And then over a monthly timeline – not days or weeks – slowly, experiment with what you can handle.

Avoid denial of CFS or the "Half and Half" dangerous approach. Don't wallow in "Oh, Woe is Me" territory. Proactively control your own Attitude and Behaviors. Ignore the negative attitudes and behaviors of others. Face depression straight-on and recognize it as a side effect of CFS that can be transformed into proactive work towards wellness. And decide to let all the negative, destructive energy go...

If you give yourself the opportunity to Be Sick and to Be a Patient, you could make steady progress toward regaining your health so that maybe you too can defeat Chronic Fatigue Syndrome.

STEP SIX
FUEL YOUR WELLNESS

I f you want to defeat Chronic Fatigue Syndrome, you need to supply your body and subsequently your immune system and biochemical pathways with the tools to self-heal and also, the supporting environment in which to succeed. This chapter is all about how to fuel your body back to wellness.

As you've heard all your life, "You are what you eat." And like most of us, you probably have a roller coaster history of intentional "healthy" eating followed by periods of regressive "unhealthy" foods. I will shamefully admit to my high school lunch of choice consisting of two cartons of milk, a small bag of potato chips and a large Ring Ding® with occasional peanut butter cravings which led to a substitution of Funny Bones®. In college I belonged to a food co-op and ate "close to the dirt" with a brief stint as a macrobiotic. Then I started a career and after long entry level hours, and a brutal commute, I consumed frozen dinners with "healthy" descriptions – as if. Then came kids and we were instilled with the need to feed them foods that were free of "contaminants" so we ate less prepared foods and more "organic" foods. When the kids grew up and discovered the "white bread" world, we slipped into kid food land and the accompanying junk foods. But those are all just excuses for not eating as we know we should.

EAT HEALTHY AND OFTEN

If you skip breakfast, eat on the run, and then grab whatever is available, you need to reassess your habits. Your immune system is trying to get things sorted out 24/7 and it needs a consistent fuel supply. From now on, you're eating three meals a day – they don't have to be huge – with smaller healthy snacks in between. This will also help you to keep a reasonable blood sugar level which can be a problem for some CFS patients.

Don't worry about making "perfect" meals. You don't have the energy to spend on constant daily food preparation. It will require some planning to make sure that you have "ready-to-eat" healthy food on hand but not much. Grocery stores are full of healthy foods. Whole wheat breads, lean deli meats, roasted chickens, humus, tabouli, low-fat yogurt and cheeses, fresh "organically grown" greens already washed in a bag, fruits (an apple a day), granola, nuts, raisins, veggies, etc. You really only have to "cook" one meal a day. So eat a moderate amount of healthy food over the course of the day and you'll be evenly fueling your wellness.

EAT POSITIVELY

So, to fuel your wellness, you need to eat well. Meaning eat healthy. Meaning eat moderately – not at the extremes. Meaning eat "positively" and avoid foods and substances that you know are negative.

You should eat lean protein, lean dairy, vegetables, fruits, nuts (unless you're allergic), legumes and whole grains. No new news here. And I'm not talking vegan either. Just normal, everyday healthy eating. And you know exactly what this is because you've been hearing about it since you were a kid. Eat like you know that you should. And don't deny yourself the occasional items that you enjoy. Just don't overindulge in them either. Again, eat moderately. If you were your immune system, what would you want to be fed when you're sick and struggling to get well? You'd want foods rich in nutrients that build you up, not empty, potentially damaging calories.

AVOID THE NEGATIVE

If you grew up in America, you've known since childhood that to be healthy you needed to eat healthy food. Which foods were "healthy" varied from cultural group to cultural group, with the influence of Madison Avenue thrown into the mix. Over time, some of that changed. But we all have a basic understanding of what is good for you and what *isn't* good for you.

When the results of a recent study made the popular press, my husband felt validated. Not only was a glass of red wine every day a good thing for your heart, a daily coffee habit increased the benefit. Talk about the Holy Grail of legal drugs! Add nicotine and you've got the Holy Trinity. As Americans, we *love* our legal drugs and we indulge daily. Sorry to break up the party but your immune system *hates* them. And not to ignore the scientific studies that have been touting the red wine/coffee connection, I'm sure that the research is thorough and well considered. But, in my opinion, when you have Chronic Fatigue Syndrome, you and your immune system are struggling to get back to a healthy state. Think about the times that you've been sick and then had a few drinks. While you were drinking, you were feeling OK. But the next morning, you were feeling worse. And your brain groaned,

"I shouldn't have drunk last night."

Have you ever read the guides to healthy living or the medicinal/herbal healing prescriptions that come from the Eastern Medicine tradition? There is a clear message that caffeine, alcohol and nicotine are substances which need to be eliminated – especially when you're sick(6). They can be, in effect, poisonous to your immune system. And these ideas don't come from the latest ten year case study or a double-blind placebo-controlled drug trial. They come out of a tradition which goes back thousands of years with an experiential knowledge base about the effect of thousands of plants and other substances on the whole human body – not just one symptom or disease. Obviously, they aren't making this recommendation on a whim or "hot" prospect. And it makes logical sense. Your immune system is struggling to get its act together - to get the biochemical pathways functioning correctly again and to operate in normal mode. Our legal drugs muddy the communication and stimulate reactions that are potentially counter productive.

So quit drinking alcohol. And if you drink caffeinated coffee or tea, switch over to decaf. It's not a permanent lifestyle change. If you smoke, don't go cold turkey – the withdrawals can be brutal. But cut back until you can cut nicotine out. You're immune system will enjoy the break and be able to focus what resources it has on dealing with CFS.

Soda is another American habit that we cherish. I always wonder when I see the ads that laud no calories, no sugar, no carbs, no caffeine. Do people ever ask themselves what actually *is in* those cans? Not one single nutrient. It's a bunch of garbage – dyes, chemical sweeteners and flavorings – that your body has to process and get rid of. Don't treat your body like a sewage treatment plant. Everything that goes into your mouth should be beneficial, not negative. What should you be drinking? Water – but more on that in Step Seven.

Avoid a lot of fats, fatty meats, sugars and additives. Avoid traditional fast food – I won't name any names. Avoid a lot of packaged foods. If you can't pronounce it, why eat it? On the other side of the issue, don't turn into an obsessive nutritionist. Find the right balance that works for you.

Avoid unnecessary over-the-counter medications that simply mask your symptoms. Work with your doctor to make sure that every drug you're taking – whether prescribed or not – is *actually* needed. In the bustle of the medical practitioner's office, it's easy to lose track of every patient's drug profile. Revisit your medications with your doctor every time you have an appointment. Make sure you're taking only what you need to support your immune system's effort to self-heal.

So eat moderately and avoid the extremes. Eliminate the "optional" drugs that muddy the biochemical pathways. And when you're making food choices, stop listening to your taste buds and your stomach, and start thinking like your immune system. Enough said.

Nutritional Supplements

For every Chronic Fatigue patient you talk with, you'll be told about a different supplement that is a "must take" to get well. Reading the CFS books – and there are many – will identify more. When searching the web, you'll find more. And more and more and more. Take them all and you'll have a two foot-long line-up of plastic bottles on your kitchen counter. When I was sick, I expended a lot of time, money and precious energy in pursuit of the magic pill. I didn't find it. Wake up to the reality that, as of this writing, there is no "silver bullet" supplement that will restore your health and leave CFS behind you. But I did ultimately settle on a sensible sampling of supplements to support the immune system and the muscles and joints which are suffering as well.

As you're probably aware, recommending supplements is a virtual mine field. For every study that supports the need for a particular supplement and its critical role in supporting, let's say immune function, there are two other studies that cast doubt on the first study. Let the scientists duke it out. Just taking a reasonable amount of daily supplements will be a solid improvement for most CFS patients and will pay off by feeding your immune system some of the things it may be missing.

If you pay attention to some of the recommended daily amounts for these supplements per the popular literature and the web, the logic often seems to be "if a little is good then a whole lot is best." I don't come from the "more is better" school of supplements. The following are reasonable amounts but follow your own instincts. Avoid mega doses. And the debate about the effectiveness of "natural" versus "synthetic" sources seems to continue. I lean toward natural but use your own judgment.

RECOMMENDED DAILY

A Multivitamin/Multimineral from a reliable source: This is the shotgun approach to cover what is missing from your diet. Most multi supplements include not only your standard Vitamins and Minerals but a whole new group of supplements that have reached "mainstream" status including selenium, Coenzyme Q10 and others – some of which have been identified as beneficial to CFS patients. Are they? Maybe.

Vitamin C – 500 mg to 1000 mg: Vitamin C (ascorbic acid) has many benefits including the support of a healthy immune system. Although the mega doses publicized by Linus Pauling are not widely supported, there is general agreement that moderate doses of C arc healthful (7).

Vitamin D – 200 IU and Calcium 500mg: Calcium is vital to bone and joint health. Vitamin D complements the absorption of calcium and current research has suggested several important functions including the maintenance of a healthy immune system (8). If you take a calcium supplement, be sure that it's combined with Vitamin D. If you drink OJ from a carton, buy one with added calcium *and vitamin D.*

Vitamin E – 400 IU: Vitamin E with antioxidant properties is important for the proper function of nerves and muscles (8). It has also been shown to play a role in immune function, in DNA repair and other metabolic processes (9).

BLUE-GREEN ALGAE

In my travels to find the elusive magic supplement that would cure my CFS, I encountered many offerings from every imaginable source. After a while, the sales spiels started to remind me of the traveling peddlers of old who sold wellness in a bottle – known as "snake oil" – with outrageous claims about its healing properties. A product looking for suckers. And yet, I was beginning to understand the people who spent their last hard earned dollar on a bottle of promises. When you're feeling desperate for a way to get your health back and your life, even a savvy consumer can be willingly duped. I tried a few of them but for the most part, I spent a lot of effort and money to get minimal effect. There was one exception.

Spirulina, or blue-green algae, is simply a one-celled alga that is found in warm, alkaline fresh water. It is about 60 percent *complete* protein, meaning that it contains all of the essential amino acids. It is rich in vitamins and minerals and is easily absorbed. Researchers have found a history of harvesting and eating spiulina in Central America since the time of the Aztecs and it is still consumed as a food source today in Central Africa (10).

From all the information I found, it seemed like a kind of new age fast food. I imagine that if the military was into health food, their MREs – Meals-Ready-to-Eat – would contain some spirulina. I decided to try it and, for me, I could feel a difference in my energy levels. Not a leap out of bed and do jumping-jacks energy, but a positive sense of improved, available energy. OK. Now, that sounds *really* academic.

If you investigate, you'll find a lot of speculation about spirulina but very little hard research (11). Bottom line for me was that it seemed like a good source of food to support my immune system and if I was going to gamble on any one of these "snake oils", I liked the odds on spirulina. I took six to eight tablets (500 mg each) per day, a few with each meal. Check it out and decide for yourself. Just for the record, I don't own any personal interest in a blue-green algae business.

FOOD ALLERGIES

As part of your initial medical evaluation and diagnosis, you should have been screened for food allergies and other GI problems that can present like Chronic Fatigue Syndrome. If not, you should investigate this with your current physician.

FUELING YOUR WELLNESS

You won't find any meal plans, recipes or daily food charts in this book. Most people know what healthy eating is, regardless of their current habits. If you need that kind of structure, there are plenty of helpful books out there. Get one and get started.

Bottom line – In order to support your immune system and feed it back to health, you should:

- Eat healthy food in moderation
- Eat three meals a day with snacks in between
- Avoid too much fat, sugar and empty calories
- Avoid alcohol, caffeine, nicotine
- Avoid heavily processed foods and fast foods
- Take daily vitamin and mineral supplements
- Drink plenty of water and avoid soda
- Take only the drugs that treat specific, crucial symptoms
- Avoid unnecessary drugs that only serve to muddy the bio-pathways

There are not any ground-breaking realizations on this list. So do what you know you should be doing. Simply put, every gasoline-powered engine has a fuel filter. It screens out the worst contaminants before the fuel reaches the engine. You need to install a fuel filter on your mouth by making intentional choices about what you are putting into it. Your immune system will benefit greatly and, in turn, you may be one step closer to defeating Chronic Fatigue Syndrome.

STEP SEVEN
MAINTAIN AN OPTIMAL BLOOD PRESSURE

An important piece in the medical mystery of Chronic Fatigue Syndrome seems to be related to blood pressure. Whether optimizing the CFS patient's blood pressure addresses one of the primary causes of CFS or treats a side effect that prolongs the illness, is unknown. For many researchers, it isn't even considered significant except for the patients who fail tilt table tests where they become dizzy when quickly raised from a horizontal to a standing position. But with so many personal success stories and case histories showing up in the literature and popular press, it's hard to ignore. Is this an issue for all, most or just some CFS patients? For me, actively managing my blood pressure at an optimal level proved to be the "frosting" on my protocol cake. So here's how the blood pressure piece fell into place for me.

THE BLOOD PRESSURE CONNECTION

Two things happened simultaneously as I left CFS behind me on my path back to full health. I was on track with the protocol and was dedicated to following it. I had progressed successfully to where I no longer had serious relapses. My only slips back were brief and kept me mindful of my daily activity levels. It was a slow but steady climb without the roller coaster. I had reached a point where I was starting to function again, not fully, but with the energy to grocery shop, or do some light cleaning without suffering a relapse. But I would sometimes have dizziness or vertigo when I got up or moved after rest or after climbing stairs accompanied with some fatigue. At this point I had come a long way but it seemed like I had "hit a wall". No matter what I did, I couldn't progress any further. And, for me, this was not acceptable. I wanted my full health back. There was to be no compromise. I wanted to defeat CFS.

I was, after all, thankful not to be chained to my bed anymore. I was still taking naps and being conservative, all of which was paying off. And I moved with confidence through each day, although I was still unable to hold down a job. But my slow, steady progress had come to a stand still.

Then my advocate, my husband, John, told me about a study that a colleague of his had sent him. Researchers in the School of Medicine at Johns Hopkins University in Baltimore had identified several Chronic Fatigue Syndrome patients who also had Neurally Mediated Hypotension (12). NMH is a condition where the body is unable to properly regulate blood pressure when a person suddenly stands or exerts energy. Normally, the body elevates blood pressure in response to exertion but, instead, with NMH the messages are miss-communicated and the opposite happens. The blood pressure drops, causing light-headedness, vertigo and sometimes fainting. This was most clearly associated with CFS patients whose blood pressure was normally low. Immediately, CFS researchers outside of Johns Hopkins were paying attention. NMH was questioned as the possible cause of Chronic Fatigue Syndrome or maybe a side effect of long term CFS. In the end, researchers settled on an "association" between the two for a subset of CFS patients (13).

This new information seemed to be a good fit for my dizziness problem. We looked into it further and, on the next visit to my doctor, I was excited about the opportunity to discuss it with him. To my delight, he had also seen the article. Given my medical profile and history – I have normally low blood pressure – he felt that NMH was an appropriate diagnosis and that we should go ahead with treatment, forgoing the actual tilt table test.

His approach for treatment was to use drugs. I subsequently tried Fludrocortisone (Florinef) and then I tried a beta blocker. Both gave me side effects of irregular heart rhythms and, generally, I just felt awful on them. I was probably on each one for less than a week before I stopped taking them.

After the drugs failed to address my low blood pressure problem, we reviewed the literature and found that drinking more water and increasing salt intake could raise my blood pressure. How? A higher blood volume would naturally elevate my blood pressure. Drinking more water would increase the available liquids and salt naturally helps you to retain water in your blood stream. At my next office visit, I discussed this with my doctor. He agreed and recommended an additional gram of sodium per day with four 8 oz glasses of water. We discussed the possible health risks but since I already had low blood pressure when resting, there would probably be no problem. I did agree to monitor my resting blood pressure for the first several months just to be sure it wasn't getting too high.

Just to clarify, the terms salt and sodium are often used interchangeably. Salt is actually sodium chloride – which is about 40 percent sodium.

I began drinking more water and adding salt to my diet and immediately realized how difficult it was for me to consume one additional gram of sodium. Half a teaspoon of salt stirred into a glass of water is tough to drink! Many prepared foods nowadays are intentionally lower in sodium and a diet of salty potato chips and snacks would quickly turn anyone into a blimp. Eventually we realized that tomato juice and tomato/vegetable juice contain a lot of sodium. An eight ounce can has almost a gram. I also discovered salt tablets which are non-prescription and are used by people who do physical labor under hot conditions where they sweat a lot. The salt tablets, about 180mg of sodium each, help them to retain fluids and avoid heat prostration.

After one month on this new regimen, *in addition to continuing with all the other steps in the protocol*, I was able to say that I was feeling better. Something that had felt "wrong" with my system for so long, was not feeling so wrong anymore. How's *that* for scientific accuracy? And the stiffness and pain in my joints and muscles was decreasing. I monitored my blood pressure, which was higher than normal for me but completely normal within the general population. After three months of this new water and salt regimen, I felt the best that I had in more than two years. I told my advocate that I felt normal and healthy again. But I was wrong because one month later, I felt even better. And I continued for six more months to think that I was fully "normal" again only to realize the following month that I was still improving. I had been sick so long that I had forgotten what a healthy system felt like.

Finally, after about eight months, I reached a point where whatever was being repaired by the water and salt regimen, was complete. After that, I was in maintenance mode. I continued to follow all the steps in the protocol and to make sure I got plenty of water and additional salt each day, but the wall that I had run into was gone. Once again, I was making upward progress.

The more my advocate and I began to think about all this new information and to think about me and my medical history, the puzzle began to fit together. Like so many people who listen to nutritionists in order to manage those aspects of their health that are within their control, I had cut back on salt because the message was that it is "bad" for you. I had virtually no salt in my diet, other than what I got from natural food sources and the limited packaged foods that I consumed. I actually preferred "no salt" snacks. And I never added salt to my cooking or to my food at the table, preferring instead to use herbs and spices. So, in essence, I created a situation where my salt intake was low. But was this a bad thing?

The human body is unable to make its own sodium and must get it from food sources. According to the institute of Medicine at the National Academy of Sciences, "Healthy 19 to 50-year-old adults should consume 1.5 grams of sodium and 2.3 grams of chloride each day – or 3.8 grams of salt – to replace the amount lost daily on average through sweat and to achieve a diet that provides sufficient amounts of other essential nutrients." (14)

So what was happening to me as I increased my daily intake of water and salt over that eight month period? Clearly the increase in my blood pressure alleviated the dizziness and fainting. But was this the lone trigger that brought on such an overall positive result? Why did I get progressively better over a long period? Did this higher blood pressure enable blood to better circulate throughout my body and reach tissues that may have been blood – and thus – food/oxygen starved? Did the higher level of salt and its accompanying minerals supply something that had been missing or in low supply? Is there a connection between my increased water and salt intake and the progressive decrease of pain and stiffness in my muscles and joints? Lots of questions...

I think the truth may lie somewhere in between. Western medicine has a tendency to see the human body in separate parts and continues that tendency into its research, which develops drugs that target specific reactions. Most of the clinical trials for CFS and NMH used drugs to test the association with Chronic Fatigue patients, not water and salt. Maybe there's a lot we have yet to understand about the way that our bodies require, absorb and process different vitamins and minerals – the combinations and complementarities. Maybe nature has some secrets yet to be revealed. For now, I'm reminded that the ocean is where we evolved. And since our bodies don't naturally produce salt, maybe we need to better understand our requirements for sodium and in what combinations with other minerals/substances that naturally occur in the ocean. My thoughts for what they are worth...

THE RESEARCH

So what answers can the scientific community contribute to these questions? Here's a sampling of results from several studies.

Orthostatic intolerance (OI) is a condition where the body fails to properly adjust to an upright position. Blood flow, heart rate, and blood pressure are involved in this malfunction. There are multiple types of OI including NMH (neurally mediated hypotension) and POTS (postural orthostatic tachycardia syndrome). There are several studies which have found a significant association between CFS patients – both adult and children – and OI (13,14,16,17,18,19,20).

Low levels of circulating blood volume and red blood cell mass have been found to be significantly associated with CFS patients (21).

Hypercoagulation (thickening) of blood in CFS patients has been associated with not enough oxygen and nutrients reaching cells – simply put, thicker blood is harder to pump and harder to pass through to tissues (22).

But of course, there are other studies that dismiss all of the above findings...

What Does It All Mean?

If you look for a trend in these studies, they all seem to dance around the subject of tissue-level access to proper blood supply and proper management of blood pressure. To me, it seems to be the other "elephant" in the Chronic Fatigue Syndrome room. Or maybe it's just too iffy, not yet proven in a clinical long-term study to risk promoting. I am a layperson and have no scientific or medical practitioner's reputation to risk. I'm just one of the unfortunates who contracted CFS but who is now fortunate to be fully healthy again. And one of the pieces to my successful recovery was to raise my blood pressure back to normal (for me) and even a bit higher. So I'm raising the question. Whatever the causes of CFS may be, and until we understand more about it, could one of the treatments – in addition to the rest of the protocol – be to naturally raise a patient's blood pressure with water and salt? Therefore, getting more blood to starved tissues and starting the patient at a higher blood pressure in order to avoid bottoming out and /or to address malfunctions which could be a result of too little sodium in the diet?

Based on what happened to me, I believe that the answer is yes. Here's my take. I have had naturally low blood pressure all of my life. This was always seen by my various doctors as a good thing. I would probably never have to worry about high blood pressure, which in the United States is a significant issue for an estimated one third of the adult population (23). Then, along came CFS. I believe that, because my blood pressure dropped even lower, I fell out of the acceptable range and began to show symptoms of dangerously low blood pressure. Subsequently, I suffered from dizziness and vertigo. And when the association between NMH and CFS patients came along, I was a match. So I was treated for NMH and, in the process of continuing the regimen for longer than was immediately necessary, I continued to get stronger and stronger over an eight-month period.

But what could this indicate for all the other CFS sufferers? Did their blood pressure drop too but it wasn't noticeable because they dropped within the range of normal? To go from a normal higher blood pressure to a normal lower blood pressure is viewed as a good thing in the medical practitioner's office. But maybe this is significant if you're suffering from CFS. And there may also be in play a disinclination for a physician who has been treating many patients for high blood pressure as a regular part of their practice, to come around to the idea that raising a patient's blood pressure could be an effective and prudent – not to mention the potential malpractice risk – course of therapy.

MANAGE YOUR BLOOD PRESSURE

So what does this mean for you? Does this apply to you? Talk to your advocate and **work with your doctor.** Explore whether or not NMH or OI may apply to you. If not, is your current resting blood pressure lower than it was before you contracted CFS? Determine, with your doctor's guidance, your optimal blood pressure level and establish a water and salt regimen to help you reach and maintain that level. Be sure to monitor your resting blood pressure to avoid raising it too high. And in keeping with the rest of the steps in the protocol, use water and salt in moderation. Mega doses are dangerous. **And only try this under your doctor's supervision.**

Continue with all the other steps in the protocol because CFS is a systemic illness. In general, make sure that you are drinking enough water. Your immune system will appreciate it. And take a look at your salt intake. You may be getting too little. **Again, review your situation and make adjustments under your doctor's care.** Managing your blood pressure may be another important step on your path if you hope to defeat Chronic Fatigue Syndrome.

STEP EIGHT
MANAGE YOUR STAGES OF RECOVERY

As diseases go, Chronic Fatigue Syndrome is not generally life threatening. But it is *lifestyle* threatening. And it is cruel the way it plays with you – physically feeling up one day and plummeting downward into exhaustion the next. In order to successfully defeat CFS, you have to work at taking the highs and lows out of the roller coaster and changing the pattern into a gradual, steady, uphill climb. This will happen over a long period – at least a year. You'll need all the patience you can gather to go the distance.

STAGES OF RECOVERY

When I was struggling with Chronic Fatigue Syndrome, I was desperately searching for clues as to how to get well again. As I pored over whatever I could find, it always amazed me to read, in source after source, that I should be getting moderate exercise every day. Suggestions included a short walk, a yoga class, twenty minutes of exercise with weights, etc. The phrase "deconditioning from lack of activity" was often discussed in the literature as a danger for CFS patients. In the first two years of my illness, this was either impossible – I didn't have the physical ability to do this – or would bring on a severe relapse after a few days. What kind of patients were they talking about?

Eventually I came to realize that there are stages of CFS and that sufferers in different stages need to hear different advice about how to get well. Depending on your level of recovery, you can only handle certain levels of physical activity. Here's a simple guideline to use to determine where you are in your recovery.

- **Always Challenged Stage** – On a daily basis, you struggle to dress, shower, navigate stairs, and generally move around without pain and exhaustion. Leaving the house is rare and never without assistance. Most of your day is spent resting or trying to sleep but you aren't successful in feeling stronger for long.

- **Usually Challenged Stage** – On a day-to-day basis, you feel alternately strong and then weak. One day you're able to sustain a physical effort of 30 minutes or so, only to be followed later by severe exhaustion the same day or the next. This physical effort is not what you would define as "exercise". Cooking a meal, doing a quick grocery shop, a *brief* walk, or working at your desk will usually do you in. But in general, you feel stronger when you're inactive.

- **Half Time Challenged Stage** – Sound Familiar? This is potentially the Most Dangerous Stage – at least it was for me. You're feeling strong enough to get through a day confident that you are better, although feeling some exhaustion. You have a couple of good days, followed by a bad day. This can be the prime stage for relapse because you can easily over estimate what you can safely handle. You can end up playing "Chutes and Ladders" as I did. CFS seems to love this stage.

- **Almost There Stage** – You're feeling consistently strong each day with occasional bouts of "that CFS feeling". You're trying to get back to your normal lifestyle which might include work, family responsibilities, etc. You're physically feeling more "normal" than you have in a long time. But not fully there yet.

Obviously, patients in each of these stages can handle completely different levels of activity. If you are successfully following the protocol, you will pass through each of these stages, hopefully from most severely sick to completely well again. For me, before we had figured out the protocol, I was in the first three stages several times, in various sequences. All of which was the result of "acting like a patient" long enough to feel better and then trying to ramp up to my old lifestyle too quickly. For me, with each relapse, my symptoms got worse.

Don't Get Anxious

Resist the desire to get back to your old lifestyle as fast as possible. Yes, everything seems to be "falling apart" in your life. Maybe finances are strained. Or your family is struggling. Or you just can't stand the snail's pace recovery anymore. This is when your determination to get your normal life back will override your best judgment about where you are in your recovery and what you can handle. This is when you must assert that part of you that understands your desire to get well *permanently*. That part of you that doesn't want to settle for "living with" CFS. That part of you that wants to get on with the rest of your life and that doesn't want CFS to be part of it.

EVALUATE YOUR READINESS OBJECTIVELY

As you progress toward wellness, you'll be constantly asking yourself – How am I doing? Should I try this? Am I ready for that? How is my recovery pace? Too fast? Too slow? When can I take on more? How will I know what I can handle? If you've been following the protocol, you already have the means to make reliable decisions about your abilities. Your Daily Record, your advocate, and your doctor will be your best litmus tests to evaluate your recovery pace and to concur or disagree with your own opinion of what you can handle.

REVIEW YOUR PATTERNS

You should see your doctor once a month. You should be reviewing your progress with your advocate weekly and probably more often. And if you're anything like me, you're staring back at yourself in the bathroom mirror every morning asking yourself what you can handle. In combination with the hard data that you can review in your Daily Record, you should have plenty of input available to help keep you successfully paced to potentially defeat CFS.

How do you balance all this input? What if you, your doctor and your advocate are not all in agreement about your pace?

My husband and I are sailors. And if you've spent any time on large bodies of water, you know that weather conditions can change radically in the space of a few minutes. One moment, you're running before the wind under full sail, in a moderate breeze, wing-on-wing, listening to the swish of the bow wave as you find that perfectly balanced groove through the water. You're reclining in the cockpit, not a single luff in the sails and life is sweet. Five minutes later, you're scrambling over the deck, your pulse doing a "riverdance", while you wrestle a large genoa down, trying to avoid being knocked silly by a sudden, uncontrolled jibe. And you wonder – how did that happen? We learned that we had set a bad pattern where one of us would look up wind and raise the question of whether or not we should shorten sail or adjust our course, and we would discuss it. Then not do anything, because we weren't in agreement. Big mistake. Finally, we learned that when one of us suggested a sail change, we did it. Right then. No hesitation. No drawn-out discussion. With CFS, we learned to adopt the same agreement.

So, working with your advocate and doctor, if one of you suggests that you're doing too much or taking on more than you can handle, change right then. Drop back a bit and stabilize. Learn to trust each other's sense of where you are in your recovery. Be sure to review your daily record and adhere to successful patterns. Try to avoid the mode where you have to get into negative territory before you recognize that you're overdoing it. And conversely, you need to be in agreement when you think you can take on a little more. It's the steady, confident progressive steps toward recovery that you want to enable, with repetition, until you have a long line of successful steps that may give you the opportunity to defeat CFS.

EXERCISE READINESS

If you are in the Always Challenged Stage or the Usually Challenged Stage, you are *not yet* ready for formal exercise. The activities that you are struggling to handle on a daily basis are enough. The risk of developing some muscle atrophy as you carefully pace yourself seems trivial when compared to the gains you're making over-all against Chronic Fatigue Syndrome. Once you're well, you can regain your muscle tone and stamina. But first, you need to get to a place where exercise is a reasonable next step and won't put you back on the negative roller coaster ride of CFS.

As you gain confidence in your readiness to approach real exercise again, remember to take it slow. A short walk is a good start. There are many exercise shows on cable TV, which you can watch and gradually work up to without an audience. And before you work with light weights, be able to consistently do all the repetitions *without* the weights. If you're experiencing dizziness, as a precaution, I usually drank a can of vegetable juice a half-hour before exercise to avoid problems.

Again, take it slow and smile as you realize just how far you've come – being ready for exercise means that you may be well on your way to defeating Chronic Fatigue Syndrome.

FOLLOW THE PROTOCOL

As you manage your Stages of Recovery, be as honest as you can about where you are along the path back to full health. And if you are serious about defeating Chronic Fatigue Syndrome – not just living with it, then you will:

Understand Your Version of CFS – Keep and review a daily record of your sleep, medications, activities and severity of symptoms. Data that is recorded cannot be muddied by your persistent "brain fog". Any format will work as long as you do it and can understand what you've written. Over time, your version of CFS will emerge in patterns. You'll want to repeat the positive ones and avoid the negative.

Find a Doctor Who Will Work with You – Someone who understands CFS. Don't be discouraged if it takes a while. Finding the right doctor is worth the effort. Once you have a doctor, work with your physician to determine the appropriate treatment plan for you. Take medications to address the most critical problems, but don't overmedicate. Remember that your biochemical pathways are malfunctioning and confused. Avoid adding more confusion. If your doctor is quick to whip out the prescription pad, ask for other alternatives. In what other ways could this symptom be treated? See your doctor regularly and bring your daily record.

Break the Cycle of Fatigue – Prioritize time for deep, rejuvenating sleep. Take the appropriate medications under your doctor's care in an environment which supports uninterrupted sleep. Eliminating the downward spiral of sleep deprivation is fundamental to defeating CFS. Once you have stabilized your sleep patterns, then you can begin the slow, steady progress toward health that will alleviate your chronic fatigue rather than add to it.

Build a Support Network – Identify and honestly work with your Advocate or whatever method of "advocacy" works best for you. Use this person – or people – as your sounding board, your connection to a support system, your advisor, your trusted companion through the frustration of CFS and your best opportunity to know what you're ready to handle through objective eyes. Maintain and use a wider support network.

Be Sick! Be a Patient! – CFS is a real disease (even if other people don't seem to think so!) and you need to treat it like one if you ever hope to be fully well again. Acting half on and half off will only keep you sick. Get used to the need to change your lifestyle – temporarily – so that you can focus on being a patient and getting healthy again.

Fuel Your Immune System – Feed your immune system healthy, positive food. Avoid the negative. Take supplements and drink plenty of water. Avoid alcohol, caffeine and nicotine.

Maintain an Optimal Blood Pressure – Under the care of your doctor, drink plenty of water and increase your sodium intake in order to support nutrition at a cellular level.

Manage Your Stages of Recovery – Patiently make slow, steady forward progress on your way to full health. Give yourself the time needed to heal. Understand the different stages of CFS recovery and establish a dialogue of trust between your Advocate, your doctor and yourself to determine what you can handle. Use the hard data in your Daily Record. And be determined to stick with the protocol.

Make a commitment to work toward regaining your full health. I'm hopeful that, like me, you'll be able to **Defeat Chronic Fatigue Syndrome – You won't have to live with it.**

BE WELL AGAIN! LIFE AFTER CFS

When I was in the depths of CFS, struggling with all the physical symptoms and the weight of my own discouragement over being sick with no recognized illness, I often thought about what it might feel like to be well again. I imagined being healthy with all the aspects of my life back in place again. And it kept me going through the ups and downs, just trying to keep my vision out in front of me like a dangling, orange carrot – bright with my future. I wanted it all back. I was determined to get it all back.

As I grew stronger again, I slowly reacquired parts of my life, a little at a time. But at some point, although I couldn't say exactly when, my vision of my healthy life changed. Not because I had given up trying to get there, but because I began to realize that the former life I led was not the Holy Grail I had created in my mind. I had not been proactively managing my former "healthy" life. My former life had been reactively managing me.

And, as much as I wanted my health back, I started to understand that my old life wasn't as "healthy" as I had envisioned. I was caught up in going through the motions of living but I was missing the actual living. And once I was fully healthy, I came to understand that my old life wasn't how I wanted to live anymore.

BORN-AGAIN HEALTHY PERSON

The term "born-again" is usually applied to people who have been reborn spiritually. Since regaining my full health, I consider myself to be a "born-again healthy person." Not in the "fire and brimstone - I've found salvation" vein. More like the "my health has been given back to me" variety.

When I was sick, I got a front row seat to knowing what it's like to be cognitively trapped in a non-functioning body. The parallel between my situation and the frustration of many of our elders and those with chronic illnesses was clear. I became painfully aware of how it feels to have a debilitating illness while your brain is still able to process what's happening. Then, I got to come back to full health. And most pointedly, that if I was lucky to live a long life, I could end up in the exact same place again. Although I would never recommend CFS just to get this perspective, it was the gift of my nightmare illness.

So I've chosen to jettison certain aspects of my pre-CFS life. I'm a Reformed Type A personality. By that I mean that I have intentionally chosen to down shift the pace of my life. And I try not to sweat every detail, not to require closure on everything, to not need to "control" outcomes. I had been missing a lot of living with my attention focused on the results. I had heard the phrases "stop to smell the roses" and "live in the moment". And prior to CFS, I would have defended my frequency of doing just that. But I wasn't. And now that I watch my children and all the ridiculous schedules that some parents put their kids on, I'm happy to have my kids come home and crash. Sometimes, we all just need to relax.

Now, I let things unfold within a framework. My favorite example of this is a potluck supper. Without any instructions other than "bring food", we usually end up with a delicious meal. And the time we had mostly desserts, it didn't kill us. Personally, I enjoyed the amusing decadence of it. I like to go for long walks because I can and because I like the slower pace. I actually notice the subtle changes of the seasons rather than speeding by in my car. I plan and plant my garden but I'm open to how it develops and have become especially fond of the surprise volunteers that nature plants there.

And I do "live in the moment" more that I've ever done before. When I hear people complain about this and that, I think how pleased I am to be standing there listening and not at home sick in bed. It reminds me not to fixate on the small stuff. I seek balance in my daily life and productivity on a limited number of activities – not the scattered approach of my prior life. Gratitude has become my companion as I interact with each day and I am nourished by the time that I spend with family and friends – even my teenagers who know better than anyone where my buttons are. And I find that I'm more open to all the possibilities around me than I've ever been before.

I also know that I wasn't the only one who was permanently affected by my struggle with CFS. My husband, John, was stretched to the breaking point, handling everything while I struggled to get well. My son, Greg, lost his healthy mom at two and a half, and took on the responsibility of looking after his "sick" mom. One day he rescued me when I was so weak that I fainted. He called his dad at work, managed to get a can of vegetable juice into me and kept his two-year-old sister out of trouble until I was functioning again. At the time, he was five years old and I was supposed to be the one taking care of him. My daughter, Carolyn, grew up always having a "sick" mom. One day, after I had defeated CFS, we were standing side-by-side in the kitchen. I smiled down at her, then bent and picked her up, balancing her on my hip. She looked at me in surprise with tears welling up in her eyes, then threw her arms around my shoulders and buried her face in my neck. "What's the matter?" I asked. When she looked back up at me, she said, "You've never picked me up before." She was four years old. Through my own tears, I promised her that I would pick her up, as long as I could, for the rest of my life. She weighs over one hundred pounds now and yesterday I gave her a piggy back ride around the kitchen. My children lost some of their childhood because their mom was "sick". We all lost several years of "normalcy". But we all gained the knowledge that we could come through something difficult together and the gratitude to appreciate my health as well as theirs. Not a bad trade off.

So if you are successful in following the protocol and defeating Chronic Fatigue Syndrome, you too will probably become a born-again healthy person. Revel in the gift! Standing on the summit of Mount Kilimanjaro in the blinding rays of a high altitude morning sun, I knew that Chronic Fatigue Syndrome was in my past. My present was full of gratitude and my future would be focused on living well.

RESOURCES

The Department of Health and Human Services

The Center for Disease Control and Prevention

1600 Clifton Rd
Atlanta, GA 30333 U.S.A.
www.cdc.gov

The CFIDS Association of America

PO Box 220398
Charlotte, NC 28222-0398
704-365-2343
www.cfids.org

The National CFIDS Foundation

103 Aletha Road
Needham, MA 02492
781- 449-3535
www.nfc-net.org

The Massachusetts CFIDS and FM Association

PO Box 690305
Quincy, MA 02269
617-471-5559

www.masscfids.org

The National Chronic Fatigue Syndrome
and Fibromyalgia Association

National Headquarters
PO Box 18426
Kansas City, MO 64133
816-737-1343

www.ncfsfa.org

REFERENCES

1. Centers for Disease Control and Prevention, "Genetic and Environmental Factors Impact CFS patients" Press Release April 2006 Department of Health and Human Services, http://www.cdc.gov/od/oc/media/pressrel/r060420.htm.

2. Centers for Disease Control and Prevention, "Chronic Fatigue Syndrome: Possible Causes" Department of Health and Human Services, http://www.cdc.gov/cfs/cfscauses.htm.

3. Susan Levine, "Immune System Gone Haywire?" The Science and Research of CFS: A special issue *CFIDS Chronicle* (2005-2006).

4. Centers for Disease Control and Prevention, "Chronic Fatigue Syndrome: Basic Facts" Department of Health and Human Services, http://www.cdc.gov/cfs/cfbasicfacts.htm.

5. SleepChannel – Your Sleep Community, "Sleep Stages" Healthcommunities.com Inc., http://www.sleepdisorderchannel.com/stages.

6. Taoism and the Taoist Arts, "Medicine and Diet" Taoist Arts, http://www.taoistarts.net/medicine.html.

7. WebMD feature archive, "The Supplement Frenzy: Which Ones Work?", WebMD http://www.webmd.com/diet/features/supplemt-frenzy.

8. Office of Dietary Supplements, NIH Clinical Center, "Dietary Supplement Fact Sheets", National Institutes of Health, http://ods.od.nih.gov/Health_Information/Vitamin_and_Mineral_Supplement_Fact_Sheets.aspx.

9. Office of Dietary Supplements, NIH Clinical Center, "Vitamin E Fact Sheet", National Institutes of Health, http://ods.od.nih.gov/factsheets/vitamine.asp.

10. Orio Ciferri, "Spirulina, the Edible Microorganism," *Microbiological Reviews* 1983 47(4) 551.

11. Shawn M. Talbott, *A Guide to Understanding Dietary Supplements* (New York: The Hawthorn Press, 2003), 638.

12. P.C. Rowe et al., "Is Neurally Mediated Hypotension an Unrecognized Cause of Chronic Fatigue?" *Lancet* 345 (1995) 623.

13. I. Bou-Holaigah et al., "The Relationship Between Neurally Mediated Hypotension and the Chronic Fatigue Syndrome," *Journal of the American Medical Association* 274 (1995) 961.

14. Institute of Medicine of the National Academies, "Dietary Reference Intakes: Water, Potassium, Sodium, Chloride, and Sulfate," National Academy of Sciences, http://www.iom.edu/CMS/3788/3969/18495.aspx.

15. H. Calkins and P.C. Rowe, "Relationship Between Chronic Fatigue Syndrome and Neurally Mediated Hypotension," *Cardiology Review* 6 (1998) 125.

16. R. Schondorf and R. Freeman, "The Importance of Orthostatic Intolerance in the Chronic Fatigue Syndrome," *American Journal of Medical Sciences* 317 (1999) 117.

17. Julian M. Stewart et al., "Orthostatic Intolerance in Adolescent Chronic Fatigue Syndrome," *Pediatrics* 103 (1999) 116.

18. David H. P. Streeten and Gunnar H. Anderson Jr., "The Role of Delayed Orthostatic Hypotension in the Pathogenesis of Chronic Fatigue," *Clinical Autonomic Research* 8 (1998) 119.

19. D.H. Streeten, D. Thomas and D.S. Bell, "The Roles of Orthostatic Hypotension, Orthostatic Tachycardia, and Subnormal Erythrocyte Volume in the Pathogenesis of the Chronic Fatigue Syndrome," *American Journal of Medical Science* 320 (2000) 1.

20. Jeanne Poole et al., "Results of Isoproterenol Tilt Table Testing in Monozygotic Twins Discordant for Chronic Fatigue Syndrome," *Archives of Internal Medicine* 160 (2000) 3461.

21. David Streeten and David Bell, "Circulating Blood Volume in Chronic Fatigue Syndrome," *Journal of Chronic Fatigue Syndrome* 4 (1998).

22. David Berg et al., "Chronic Fatigue Syndrome &/or Fibromyalgia As a Variation of Antiphospholipid Antibody Syndrome (APS): An Explanatory Model and Approach to Laboratory Diagnosis," *Blood Coagulation and Fibrinolysis* 10 (1999) 435.

23. American Heart Association, "High Blood Pressure Statistics," American Heart Association, http://www.americanheart.org/presenter.jhtml?identifier=4621.

ABOUT THE AUTHOR

Martha E. Kilcoyne, M.P.H., has worked professionally
in the healthcare software industry as a writer and
manager of technical support. Since recovering from
Chronic Fatigue Syndrome, she's been a full-time
mom and writer. She lives in Massachusetts with her
husband, John, their two children, Greg and Carolyn,
and two cats.

For more information about this book:
www.defeatCFS.net
Or e-mail: info@defeatCFS.net

To contact the author: Martha@defeatCFS.net

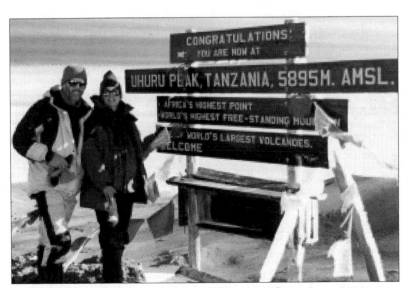

Martha and John at the summit of Mount Kilimanjaro, 2000